Tibetan Yoga of Movement

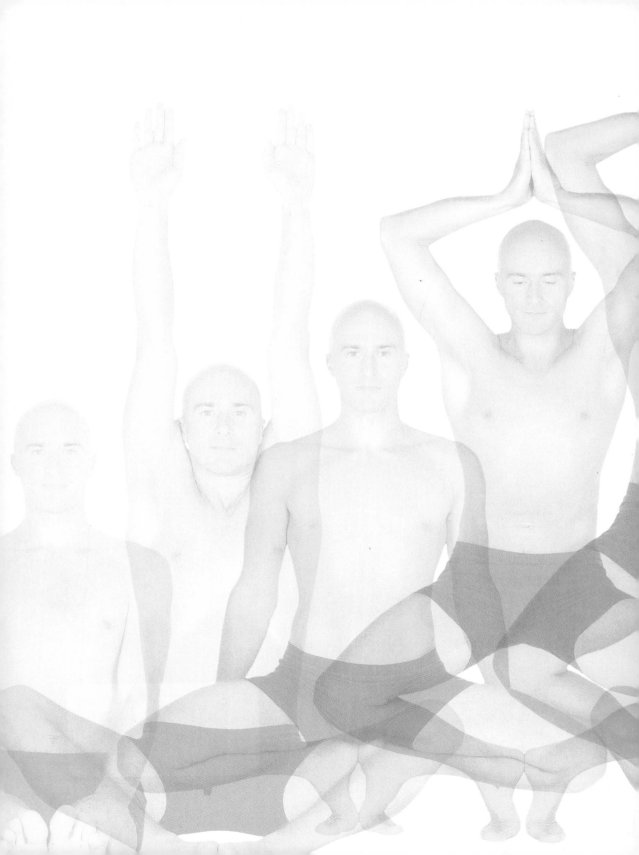

Chögyal Namkhai Norbu
& Fabio Andrico

Tibetan Yoga of Movement

The Art and Practice of Yantra Yoga

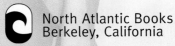
North Atlantic Books
Berkeley, California

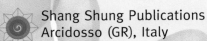
Shang Shung Publications
Arcidosso (GR), Italy

Published by

North Atlantic Books   and   Shang Shung Publications
P.O. Box 12327   Località Merigar
Berkeley, California 94712   58031 Arcidosso (GR), Italy
www.northatlanticbooks.com   www.shangshungpublications.org

Cover design by Drolma Bai
Cover photography by Kirill Ivanov
Book design by Daniel Zegunis
Photography by Ievgen Kryshen, Matthew Williams, Alison Sam, Kirill Ivanov, and David Serni
Photograph of Chögyal Namkhai Norbu by Paolo Fassoli
Photograph of Fabio Andrico by Alison Sam
Printed in the United States of America

MEDICAL DISCLAIMER: The following information is intended for general information purposes only. Individuals should always see their health care provider before administering any suggestions made in this book. Any application of the material set forth in the following pages is at the reader's discretion and is his or her sole responsibility.

Tibetan Yoga of Movement: The Art and Practice of Yantra Yoga is sponsored by the Society for the Study of Native Arts and Sciences, a nonprofit educational corporation whose goals are to develop an educational and cross-cultural perspective linking various scientific, social, and artistic fields; to nurture a holistic view of arts, sciences, humanities, and healing; and to publish and distribute literature on the relationship of mind, body, and nature.

North Atlantic Books' publications are available through most bookstores. For further information, visit our website at www.northatlanticbooks.com or call 800-733-3000.

Library of Congress Cataloging-in-Publication Data
Namkhai Norbu, 1938–
Tibetan yoga of movement : the art and practice of yantra yoga / Chögyal Namkhai Norbu, Fabio Andrico.
  pages cm
ISBN 978-1-58394-556-8
1. Yantra yoga. I. Andrico, Fabio, 1951- II. Title.
RA781.72.N36 2012
613.7'046—dc23
                    2012037651

1 2 3 4 5 6 7 8 9 Sheridan 17 16 15 14 13

IPC - 731EN12 - Approved by the International Publications Committee of the Dzogchen Community founded by Chögyal Namkhai Norbu

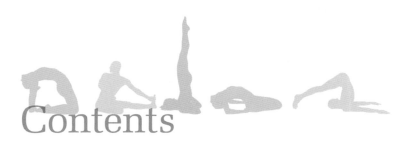

Contents

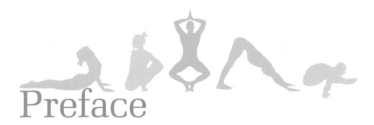

Preface

WHEN I LEARNED Yantra Yoga from my uncle, the great yogi Ugyen Tendzin, I did not know I would come to the West to teach the path of Dzogchen and Yantra Yoga to people living in a world that is so different from my homeland in so many ways. But despite the differences between East and West, we are all human beings and we all have body, energy, and mind. After arriving in Italy in the early 1960s, the first thing I taught was Yantra Yoga, a sacred and secret practice in Tibet. I decided to teach it because people asked me to, but especially because I understood how beneficial it could be for so many people to be able to have a path to real evolution.

A practice that helps coordinate body, energy, and mind while making us more balanced and free from tension is immensely important. When we have a more relaxed mind, it is possible to have a better, more harmonious, and healthy life. This is why I decided to teach Yantra Yoga: it is something anyone can find beneficial, and it can bring more compassion and understanding among people. When we are happier, we are more open to everyone and everything around us. In today's world we really need to find ways to be more relaxed and have less stress and tension so that we can experience genuine happiness and joy.

This book presents what we call the Open Level of Yantra Yoga and covers the basic practice of Yantra that anyone can apply with a little training and good will. This is my intention and my hope in opening Yantra Yoga to the world.

Chögyal Namkhai Norbu

Preface and Acknowledgments

THIS BOOK WAS written in response to the need for a comprehensive guide to the Basic Level of Yantra Yoga. It is based on the translation from Tibetan of the original eighth-century instructions for Yantra Yoga and Chögyal Namkhai Norbu's extensive commentary, first published in 2008 as *Yantra Yoga: The Tibetan Yoga of Movement*. Translated and edited by Adriano Clemente, the earlier book remains an important resource for the subtler principles of the practice as originally transmitted in an unbroken lineage since it was first recorded by Vairochana. Any shortcomings in this book or misinterpretation of the original text should be attributed to me and certainly not to Chögyal Namkhai Norbu or Adriano Clemente.

The practice of Yantra Yoga is not some recent invention proposed as an interesting set of exercises for training the body. It is a very ancient tradition steeped in Tibetan culture and the historical heritage of countless generations of spiritual practice, informed by the knowledge of the interdependence of the energies governing our inner dimension and what we perceive as the external dimension—the world around us. Ultimately, the final purpose of the practice is to help us abide in our natural condition of peace and harmony.

Yantra Yoga's benefits are far more than physical. Because its unique use of movement helps us coordinate the way we breathe and thus harmonizes and strengthens our subtle energies and vital force, it is an extremely valuable tool for any human being, not only for yoga adepts. As soon as I started to learn and practice Yantra Yoga, I realized how powerful the integration of breathing and the different holds can be, and how effectively this integration brings the practice to another level, where the movement, breathing, and positions work together in a marvelous synergy and grace.

More and more people have been discovering the benefits of Tibetan Yantra Yoga in recent years, and as the circles widen, so does the context in which they approach it. This book deliberately focuses on the aspects of the practice that are readily accessible to everyone, independent of their views, ideals, aspirations and capacities. For those interested in the spiritual aspects of the practice of Yantra Yoga, its deeper dimension cannot be conveyed by books or words alone and can only be discovered by entering the path of Dzogchen with the guidance of a qualified teacher. Also known as Total Perfection or Ati Yoga, Dzogchen is a method for recognizing our real condition. It is not a philosophical theory created by intellectual analysis, but rather an experience of direct awareness. Yantra Yoga directly supports the achievement of the authentic relaxation of body, energy, and mind so vital to this experience, and as such is closely tied to the teachings of Dzogchen.

In keeping with Chögyal Namkhai Norbu's conviction to openly share the fundamental aspects of the practice, this book covers all of the fundamental Yantra Yoga exercises. It also provides clarifications for their practical application drawn from four decades of teaching Yantra in the West. Suggested modifications are given to facilitate aspects that may be difficult to perform.

In addition to the core focus—a step-by-step guide to all of the preliminary movements and Yantras specific to this method of Tibetan yoga—we have included a section with some simple but effective warm-up exercises that you can use at the beginning of each session. Beyond easing the body into the practice of Yantra Yoga, these warm-ups are designed to help make the joints more flexible while assuring the correct position and alignment of the spine, which is paramount for performing the movements and for the smooth and harmonious flow of breathing. Appendix 1 features an extensive selection of warm-ups to complement your Yantra Yoga practice. This section also identifies specific focuses of each exercise, including the corresponding Yantras that they help train.

As explained in the introduction, one of the unique features of Yantra Yoga is that it takes into account the left and right reversal of subtle energies in female and male bodies. This is why, in the asymmetrical poses, the individual genders start the movements on opposite sides. Although it may be cumbersome for some of the more complicated positions, we have chosen to present the instructions for those Yantras gender-neutrally in the main descriptions, with gender-specific left and right directions in italics below. The italicized instructions also include practice tips and modifications.

Finally, we have included listings of the health benefits associated with each of the Yantras, many of which are based on the Tibetan understanding of the connection between the body and the elements. The overview and discussion of the basic principles of Tibetan medicine in the introduction and Appendix 3 are meant to shed light in this area.

This book was a truly collaborative effort spanning several continents, guided and inspired by our teacher, Chögyal Namkhai Norbu. By sharing his vast and unmatched knowledge of the ancient practice of Yantra Yoga, he has enriched the lives of thousands of people all over the world.

Without doubt, Chögyal Namkhai Norbu has been the most important influence in my own life as a human being, practitioner, and instructor; no words can express my profound gratitude.

I am also deeply grateful to Khyentse Yeshe, Chögyal Namkhai Norbu's son, for having shown with his actions and his teachings the importance of opening the knowledge of Yantra Yoga to the world.

Chögyal Namkhai Norbu's and Khyentse Yeshe's tireless efforts for the benefit of others motivated the generosity and enthusiasm of the many people who contributed to this book.

The practitioners who modeled for the photos, each of them exceptionally skilled in the practice of Yantra Yoga and some of them certified Yantra Yoga and Hatha Yoga teachers, gave long hours of their time until we arrived at the results we were looking for; so did the photographers.

In the collaborative spirit of the making of this book, the models come from different places around the world: Maxim Leshchenko and Alina Kramina are from the Ukraine while Katerina Stepanova is from Saint Peterburg in Russia. Carolina Mingolla is from Argentina and Nataly Nitsche Di Gennaro from Costa Rica. Each of them did their very best in accurately demonstrating the sequences of movement. The photo sessions took place in various locations with various photographers: in Kiev with Ievgen Kryshen, in New York with Matthew Williams assisted by Eliane Diallo, in Saint Petersburg with Kirill Ivanov, in Mexico City with Alison Sam, and on Tenerife in the Canary Islands with David Serni. I want to sincerely thank all of them for the time and work they dedicated to this project.

Other important contributions were made by Paula Barry and Naomi Zeitz, who participated in the process of structuring and revising the manuscript in the early stages. Additionally, Naomi coordinated the New York photo shoot and Paula provided invaluable assistance consulting the designer in the final layout phase. Anastasia McGhee helped hone the final points of the manuscript. Laura Evangelisti generously shared her in-depth knowledge of Yantra Yoga by checking the text in various stages of production, and with Tiziana Gottardi assisted in the painstaking process of sorting and reviewing the photos to ensure they correctly depict each phase of the various sequences. Dr. Phuntsog Wangmo, Elio Guarisco, and Dr. Gino Vitiello contributed their expertise to clarify and make accessible the profound knowledge of the integration between Yantra Yoga and Tibetan medicine. Artur Skura provided general assistance and coordination. Olga Bondareva and Anastasia Ermilova meticulously tweaked hundreds of images to arrive at optimum quality standards. I would like to sincerely thank all of them for the time and work they have dedicated.

Last but not least, I want to thank Dan Zegunis and Susan Schwarz: Dan was in charge of design and layout, willingly immersing himself for months in a maze of images and words and taking on the gargantuan task of bringing them together in a beautiful and effective final design. Susan was the main editor and coordinator, and though the project turned out to be much more involved than any of us anticipated, she was always there, always working hard to make it happen. The book could not have been completed without them.

One last mention goes to Natalia Pavchinskaya, who has repeatedly supported many different activities relating to Yantra Yoga, and Kirill Shilov, who helped raise funds for the book.

In closing, on behalf of everyone who participated in this project, I would like to express our deep gratitude for the opportunity to contribute to Chögyal Namkai Norbu's boundless efforts to keep Tibetan culture alive by integrating this precious ancient heritage in our day-to-day experience of the contemporary world. It is our sincere wish that despite these difficult times, the traditions and knowledge of the Tibetan people will survive and thrive for hundreds of generations to come.

Fabio Andrico

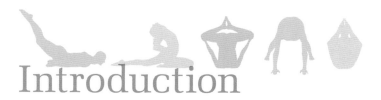

Introduction

What Is Yantra Yoga?

Yantra Yoga is a highly evolved method of movement and breathing that has been preserved in its original and unadulterated form since the eighth century, when it was first brought to Tibet by Padmasambhava, the great and legendary master who introduced Buddhism to that vast and remote kingdom. He is said to have received the instructions from the *mahasiddha* Humkara, a guru he had encountered in Nepal during his extensive travels from the land of Oddiyana throughout the Himalayan region. Later, when Padmasambhava went to Tibet, he transmitted the principles of Yantra Yoga to the scholar, master, and translator Vairochana, who in turn recorded the oral instructions in a text called *Nyida khajor* in Tibetan, The Union of the Sun and Moon.

This short and concise text is the oldest known document relating to yoga in the Tibetan Buddhist tradition. It includes a brief description of seventy-five positions similar to those of Hatha Yoga in form, but different in the dynamics of the way in which they are practiced, and especially in the coordination of movement and breathing. What is particularly remarkable about the Union of the Sun and Moon, however, is that it provides instructions on eighteen preliminary exercises, divided into three groups, that are entirely unlike any taught in Indian systems. We can only speculate where these instructions originated. But one thing we know for sure, and can recognize experientially, is that these three groups of exercises are tightly linked with the main practice. Their purposes are to warm up the body; train the different aspects of the breathing, in particular the holds; and open the energy channels. It is also interesting to note that the word *hatha* is composed of the two syllables *ha* and *tha,* meaning "sun" and "moon" in traditional Sanskrit etymology, while the Sanskrit term *yoga* is commonly translated as "union." So in effect, *Nyida* (sun and moon) *khajor* (union) embodies the same metaphor as Hatha Yoga.

In Buddhist and Hindu traditions, those two celestial bodies, so influential for planet earth, symbolize the feminine and masculine aspects of our subtle bodies, and in cultures all over the world they are associated with the male and female principles. In this context, one of the distinguishing characteristics of Yantra Yoga is that its asymmetrical poses start on alternate sides for men and women. This is because it draws on the theory that the solar and lunar energies flow on opposite sides in each gender. The reversal is a means to enhance and balance the qualities naturally present in each of us.

Another etymological clue about the underlying principle of this practice is supplied by the Sanskrit term *yantra*. It literally means "instrument" or "machine," but commonly refers to a geometric figure whose shape is considered a suitable instrument or medium to provoke a meditative experience. In the context of Yantra Yoga, it mainly refers to the movement of the body; Yantra Yoga is a vehicle that uses movement to deepen our knowledge of our real nature. In fact, while the Sanskrit term *yoga* means "union," the Tibetan translation of the term, *naljor*, more specifically refers to possessing the real knowledge of our spontaneously natural condition and being concretely in that knowledge.

Yantra Yoga, for centuries a closely guarded secret reserved for advanced yogic practitioners, was first introduced to the West in the 1970s by one of the foremost Dzogchen masters of our time, Chögyal Namkhai Norbu. He received these teachings in Tibet at a young age from his uncle Togden Ugyen Tendzin (1888–1962) and received further clarification from other contemporary masters. To preserve this knowledge, Chögyal Namkhai Norbu wrote a commentary on Vairochana's original text that has since been published in numerous languages. Thanks to Chögyal Namkhai Norbu, the lineage of Yantra Yoga remains unbroken, and we have access throughout the world to the vast and profound knowledge of this system and to the principles underlying the art of practicing it correctly. His decision to make it openly available was a direct response to the exigency of our times. Yantra Yoga courses are taught on six continents by teachers selected through a training program specifically designed by Chögyal Namkhai Norbu. His intention is to insure that the transmission of these extraordinary teachings is maintained in such a way that generations to come can enjoy the full benefits of the practice.

The Uniqueness of Yantra Yoga

Yantra Yoga is designed to coordinate our energy through the synergy of breathing and movement. As a consequence, we become healthier and able to experience a more harmonious and relaxed state of mind. We all have three aspects of human existence in common: body, energy, and mind. When we master our energy by working with our movements and breath, the body becomes flexible and strong and our mind more alert and clear, yet harmonious and relaxed.

Yantra Yoga is more than a collection of positions: each Yantra consists of a sequence of seven phases of movement and breathing centering on specific retentions of the breath. This also constitutes one of the most pronounced differences between Yantra Yoga and Hatha Yoga. While Hatha emphasizes static forms, in Yantra we do not hold asanas for a long time; the pose is just a moment in the sequence of movements defined by the respiratory rhythm and the application of one of the five types of retention of breath. In each of the seven breathing cycles of each Yantra, the inhalation, exhalation, or retention of the breath is coordinated with the rhythm, usually to a count of four. Each Yantra has a central position that explicitly facilitates one of the five types of hold. These holds—open, directed, closed, contracted, and empty—each have a precise effect on the functioning of our *prana* energy and the five elements.

Another unique feature of Yantra Yoga is that the asymmetrical poses start on opposite sides of the body for women and men. Since Yantra takes subtle energetic differences between the genders into account, the efficacy of the practice is further enhanced. As mentioned earlier, the symbolism of the sun and the moon refers to female and male energy. It is important to note here that in the Himalayan tradition of Buddhism, the male quality is lunar while the female quality is solar, a reversal of the Hindu tantric traditions, where male energy is generally identified as solar and female as lunar. In Vairochana's Yantra Yoga, the solar side is on the right for women and on the left for men, and the goal is to equalize and balance these two energies, consequently neutralizing the effect of confusion and agitation so prevalent in our fast-paced society.

Basic Principles of Tibetan Medicine

In our ordinary lives it is difficult to have concrete knowledge of the energy dimension of the body, much less know how to intervene on this level. We can, however, learn to control our breathing. In fact, by coordinating the inflow and outflow of breath with the body positions of Yantra Yoga, we are able to balance specific functions of the prana. To better understand how Yantra Yoga is able to produce beneficial effects, it is useful to have a basic idea of some of the key principles of Tibetan medicine.

According to this ancient system, which dates back at least four millennia, the universe is composed of tiny particles that each contain the qualities and functions of the four elements—earth, water, fire, and air—interacting in the dimension of the fifth element, space. In the physical body, the earth element corresponds to the flesh and bones; the water element to blood, lymph, and serum; the fire element to bodily heat; the air element to breathing; and the space element to the functions of the mind.

Tibetan medicine identifies three humors, or energies, that arise from various combinations of the elements and form the basis for the functioning of the human body. Air and space combine to form wind energy, fire and water make bile energy, and water and earth produce phlegm energy. These three energies are equivalent to the Ayurvedic principles of *vata, pitta,* and *kapha.* When they are in balance and in proper relationship to each other, we have a perfect state of health. If they are imbalanced, in excess or deficit, or abnormal in their interaction with each other, we experience disorders and diseases. In addition to these energies, the proper function of all the systems of the body is further dependent on five main pranas or winds:

1. The life-sustaining prana moves within the head and thorax and in the channels of the sense organs. It controls the functions of breathing, swallowing, sneezing, coughing, and so on. It gives clarity to the mind and the organs of the senses and allows the formation of consciousnesses.
2. The ascending prana circulates throughout the tongue, nose, and throat and into the channels of the senses. Its function is to control speech and the functioning of the memory. It presides over strength and courage.
3. The pervasive prana circulates throughout the body, mainly through the blood vessels and sensory nerves. It presides over blood circulation, hormonal secretions, development of the body, joint movement, and proper functioning of the orifices.
4. The fire-accompanying prana resides in the stomach and bowels. It presides over the digestive functions, the separation of nutrients from waste, and the assimilation of nutrients.
5. The downward-clearing prana is located in the pelvic region and circulates in the lower organs. It controls the production and emission of semen and menstrual fluids, the expulsion of feces and urine, and the process of childbirth.

Having a basic knowledge of these five winds or pranas can help Yantra Yoga practitioners understand how, through proper control of the breath in coordination with the movements of the Yantras, the practice can act to produce its benefits. These benefits not only extend to a physical level but to the energetic and mental level as well. In fact, on a more advanced level, Yantra Yoga is considered a true and complete spiritual path.

While Yantra Yoga works on the concrete level of our physical body and the subtle level of the five elements, it also teaches us how to coordinate, deepen, and relax our breathing and the prana energy associated with it. The energy can then flow through our subtle channels in a harmonious and relaxed way. We no longer need to engage in patterns of behavior that create illness. Yantra Yoga has the capacity to reverse or reduce all kinds of chronic health problems by working directly with the muscles, joints, nerves, and organs as well as with the subtle energies to create optimum health and ultimately a healthy and relaxed state of mind that gives us the ability to find ourselves in our real nature.

The Practice
of Yantra Yoga

YANTRA YOGA CAN benefit anyone who has the desire to apply its principles. It is not only for expert practitioners of yoga, but for anyone—young or old, thin or not, flexible or not so flexible. Learning to coordinate the movements with the specific rhythm of the inhalations, exhalations, and retentions will bring you a wonderful and fruitful practice of Yantra Yoga, even if you need to adapt the positions to your capacity. Regular practice will make a tangible difference in the day-to-day functioning of your body, and you will experience significant improvements in your health, energy, and ability to find a more relaxed and happy existence and overall quality of life.

The traditional Yantra Yoga sequence is a full practice in itself and includes a group of exercises designed to loosen the various joints of the body. This is the purpose of the first of the three preliminary series, called Tsigjong. Still, it is helpful to start your session with some additional warm-ups to enhance your flexibility and consequently protect your body. A selection of warm-ups designed to support your practice of Yantra Yoga has been included in Appendix 1. The warm-ups should be done according to your needs, time, and capacity. When you know which Yantras you want to practice in your session, you can also select specific warm-ups to help you prepare for those

Yantras. Correspondences between the warm-up exercises and individual Yantras have been provided in Appendix 1.

Find a nice, spacious, clean place for practicing. You will need a yoga mat, preferably the thicker kind, or a densely woven rug about the size of a mat. If you find cushions helpful, experiment with various kinds to find the one most suited to your needs. Look for something firm and resilient to give you optimum support. Props such as yoga blocks can also be useful. Wear comfortable clothing to perform the movements. Try to practice some time away from food—when you are neither in the process of digesting your last meal nor thinking about the next one—and away from the distraction of physiological needs.

A typical full-length session of Yantra Yoga consists of fifteen to twenty minutes of preliminary warm-ups, followed by the actual practice of Yantra Yoga: the Nine Purification Breathings, the three groups of preliminary exercises (Tsigjong, Lungsang, and Tsadul), at least one of the five Yantra series, a *pranayama* exercise such as Rhythmic Breathing, and, finally, the Vajra Wave. But even a session as short as seven minutes can bring tremendous benefit to your body and mind.

A number of systems of yoga advise us to approach breathing exercises with great caution. This is sound advice. We should not take powerful breathing exercises lightly, especially where we hold our breath and influence the functions of our vital energy. Never force or strain your body or your breathing. Instead, rely on consistency and training to advance in your practice, with a focused yet relaxed attitude. Be aware of your condition and possible limitations and do not overdo it. Instead of trying to overcome limitations by forcing things, use training as a tool for development and progress. Presence and awareness are the best means to prevent any possible strain in your physical or energetic condition that may result from distractedly overdoing your practice. Consult an authorized physician if you have a medical condition or any doubt about doing certain exercises. Needless to say, if you are pregnant, special care must be taken with all physical exercises, and it is crucial to consult a professional if you intend to continue your Yantra Yoga practice while carrying a child. Also, when menstruating, it is generally advisable to avoid inverted positions like the Flame, Trident, and Sword. Similarly, you may not want to perform strong closed holds at this time of the month and consciously apply them with less intensity.

Presence, not being distracted, is of paramount importance in practicing Yantra Yoga, and in turn, practicing Yantra Yoga allows us to more easily find a state of presence. When we are distracted, we are more likely to get injured. This is not only true of practicing yoga, but of any other activity as well, like driving a car or simply walking down a staircase or making a salad. Being undistracted and aware is the best protection against forcing and straining your body. If you are relaxed and aware while doing Yantra, focusing on the breathing and movements without distraction, you will enjoy safe and effective practice.

Another important and essential aspect of the practice of any kind of yoga is alignment. Everyone tries to find alignment, and rightly so. In Yantra Yoga, we not only consider the aspect of structural, anatomical alignment but also the effect of the strong influence and power exerted by our subtle energies on the movements and the positions. By practicing the five holds, we coordinate the various aspects and functions of the prana energy as well as the interaction with the energy of the five elements. When you understand how to harmoniously arrive at this kind of physical and energetic balance, your body, energy, and mind will be in a state of integrated alignment. This kind of alignment is not a generalized, mechanical alignment based on preconceived notions looking from the outside in, but rather your own natural and spontaneous alignment, the inherent harmony that is the core of our existence.

You do not have to dedicate your entire life to the practice of Yantra Yoga or to having a perfect, supple body. Anyone practicing according to their time and capacity can achieve and enjoy great benefits from this practice. Because Yantra Yoga is made up of individual groups and series of exercises, once you are familiar with the basic sequences, you will be able to put together routines on your own to suit your inclinations and schedule. Keeping a few pointers in mind, you will easily understand the various elements that can or should be included in a given session. You can also refer to the list of suggested short routines in Appendix 2.

Just as the individual exercises are composed of distinct phases of breathing and movement, each session of practice is also composed of several distinct phases. The three groups of preliminary movements (Tsigjong, Lungsang, and Tsadul) help warm up the body, train the breathing, and balance the energy. Many options are available for shortening the practice, depending on how much time you can dedicate to a session. For example, you can shorten the individual groups by doing each movement only once. Also, you can do only one or two of the preliminary groups rather than all three. Similarly, among the five series, you can include any number of groups of five in your session, and you can create a sequence composed of Yantras from any of the five series, but the order of progression should always be the same: open hold, directed hold, closed hold, contracted hold, and empty hold. After each group or series, you can either lie down and relax briefly or simply continue without interruption. The Rhythmic Breathing pranayama exercise can also be included at any point between groups or series. A final sequence of movements, the Vajra Wave, serves to correct any errors or imbalances that may have occurred as a consequence of moving or breathing incorrectly.

The best way to approach the practice is to allow the breathing to help movement and posture while allowing the posture and movement to help the breathing. As a consequence of this mutual interaction and synergy, breathing, posture, and movement evolve together, harmonizing and enriching each other and facilitating a better, more wholesome and natural condition. Practicing yoga is not about creating something new and different but about freeing ourselves from obstacles and limitations so we can find our true and natural condition. A book cannot possibly cover all of the potential imperfections that might arise when we perform movements, nor is it possible to provide in-depth advice on developing to your full capacity. For that kind of individualized guidance, you need to study directly with a qualified Yantra Yoga instructor authorized by Chögyal Namkhai Norbu or the Shang Shung Institute. Nevertheless, it is important to understand that ultimately you will always be the one truly responsible for your practice. Only you are in the dimension of your body, energy, and mind. Anything you do will be shaped by that. As much as we all try to practice as precisely as possible, making an effort to understand all the instructions and apply them correctly, in the end any Yantra you do will always be different from anyone else's. It will also be your unique experience.

Through that experience alone you will recognize the value of your practice and of this profound method. Practicing yoga is not about trying to copy a form or shape; it should be a transforming experience. If we want our body to benefit from the practice of Yantra Yoga, we have to work with our energy. The effect on our body and health will then be deeper and longer-lasting. Coordinating and freeing our energy has a much more profound ability to help us obtain good health and fitness than physical fitness exercises alone. When you have this understanding, even if your positions are not perfect and you have to adapt them to fit your capacities, the main purpose of the practice will come to fruition, and you will be able to experience and enjoy the full potential of the strength and harmony of Yantra Yoga.

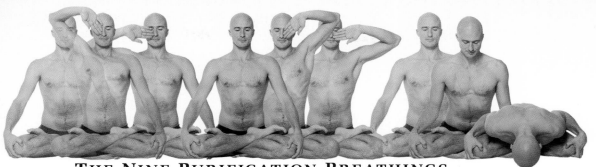

THE NINE PURIFICATION BREATHINGS

Exhaling
the Stale Air

THE ACTUAL SESSION of the practice of Yantra Yoga begins with a breathing exercise called the Nine Purification Breathings. This is an extremely effective method for exhaling stale air. Its purpose is to purify the function of our prana life force and coordinate and expand the capacity of our breathing in a correct, relaxed way. Without training, our breathing tends to be contracted and fragmented and loses its natural harmony. This can create an imbalance in our life energy, but we can purify and correct this negative condition if we make a conscious effort. The Nine Purification Breathings also serves as a short standalone practice. You can do it in the morning to tune up your energy as you start the new day. Like any other Yantra Yoga exercise, three fundamental aspects need to be taken into consideration here: the body, the breathing, and the mind, or in other words, the correct position and movement, the mode of breathing and holding, and the state of relaxed concentration.

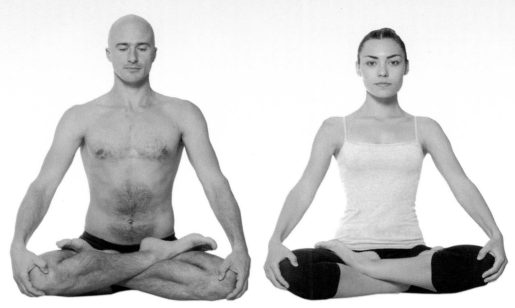

THE BODY

Sit comfortably but alert in the Vairochana position, a classic meditation position defined by seven characteristics.

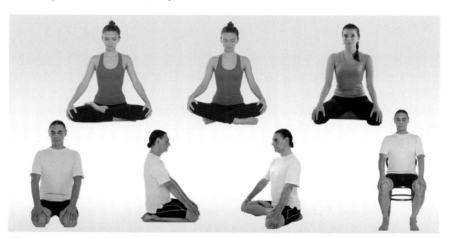

If you cannot sit in lotus, you can sit in half lotus or simply sit with your legs crossed in a comfortable way. You can also kneel, sitting on your heels with your knees closed or open. The most important factor is to have your back and spine straight. You may need to sit on a cushion to align your back, or even on a firm chair.

One method to quickly ensure that your spine is correctly aligned is to inhale, extending your arms straight up and opening your shoulders and chest well, and then exhale, lowering your hands to your knees while keeping your sides and torso stretched.

THE VAIROCHANA POSITION

1. The **back** is straight, the chin is pulled slightly in, and the nose is aligned with the navel so as to correctly align the entire spine.
2. Ideally the **legs** are crossed in the lotus position: first placing the right foot on the left thigh and then the left foot on the right thigh; the order is reversed for men.

   See "The Body" above for several alternatives to the lotus position.
3. The **hands** are on the knees pressing the thumb and ring finger in the indentations on either side of the knee.
4. The **tongue** rests on the palate behind the upper teeth. This harmonizes the fire (tongue) and water (palate) elements in the body.
5. The **eyes**, **lips**, and **teeth** are naturally closed.

   The eyes may also be half closed or open. It is important that you feel relaxed and comfortable.
6. The **chest** and **shoulders** are open.
7. The **body** is relaxed and at the same time controlled with presence.

THE BREATHING

Focus on making your inhalation and exhalation long and direct, the term used in Yantra to describe smooth and calm breathing, without any blockage or constriction in the throat. In contrast, when we breathe indirectly, our glottis is constricted and the breathing produces a distinct sound. Yantra Yoga uses the terms *direct breathing* and *indirect breathing* to make a distinction between smooth, free breathing and a deliberately constricted type of breathing specified for certain pranayamas. However, with the exception of the Tsadul pranayama and the more advanced stages of Rhythmic Breathing, all of the movements covered in this book are done with direct, smooth inhalations and exhalations, so whenever you notice that your breathing has inadvertently become indirect, relax and bring it back to direct breathing.

When inhaling, fill the lungs gradually from the bottom to the top, as if filling a vase with water. When exhaling, empty the top of the lungs first and the lower part of the lungs last. It is crucially important to exhale correctly and fully to truly benefit from the potential of the Nine Purification Breathings to expel stale air. Let your inhalation and exhalation be inspired by the shape of a grain of barley, slender at each end and thicker, fuller, in the middle. So begin inhaling and exhaling lightly, then increase the flow, and then diminish it at the end.

THE MIND

The mind is present, relaxed, alert, and focused on the flow of the breathing and movement.

THE PRACTICE

To begin the exercise, inhale slowly, directly, and completely while raising one arm, stretching your elbow upward, and opening your chest fully as you bring your hand toward your nostrils and complete the inhalation.

Women start by raising the left arm; men start by raising the right arm.

With your palm facing outward, close the nostril with your middle and ring fingers, keeping your elbow raised at the same time. Now begin to exhale in the shape of a barley grain, starting slowly then expelling most of the air and finishing slowly and softly. The exhalation should be direct and complete, from top to bottom. Naturally let your stretched elbow relax and continue to keep the nostril closed.

Then, remaining empty and without tension, return your hand to your knee and pause for a brief instant, still empty.

Repeat the same movement on the other side, raising your other arm as you inhale slowly and completely and closing the nostril with your middle and ring fingers as you exhale from top to bottom. Remaining empty, return your hand to your knee. Alternate sides until you have inhaled and exhaled three times on each side.

On the seventh inhalation, keep your hands on your knees as you inhale slowly, directly, and completely. Then, at first remaining stable and without moving, begin to exhale the upper air.

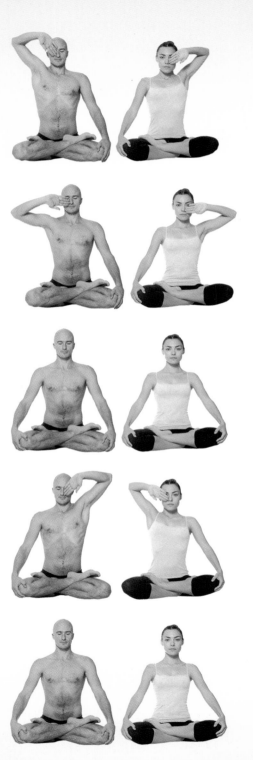

Maintaining a smooth flow, continue to exhale from the top down while bending forward. Keep your back aligned and straight and your elbows close to the body as you bend forward to completely exhale the stale air.

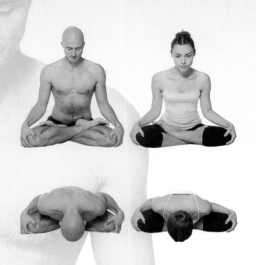

If you can, finish the exhalation with your forehead touching the floor. Otherwise, bend forward as far as you are able while keeping your back straight. Rest for just a moment, pausing your breath before inhaling and gradually rising back up to the starting position.

Expand your chest well, slowly and fully filling it with air from the bottom to the top, finishing the inhalation when you are fully upright again. Repeat this phase for a total of three times to complete all nine phases of the Nine Purification Breathings.

Applying this method will help you purify, coordinate, and harmonize your breathing and your energy. As a consequence, your mind can more easily relax in its natural condition and be present and alert. You will be less distracted and conditioned by thoughts and worries.

If you do not have much time, you can also perform this wonderfully helpful breathing exercise only three times, one time on each side and one time bending forward. It takes just a couple of minutes, but it is a highly effective method to relax and clear your mind.

COMMON MISTAKES
- *Not keeping the spine in correct alignment*
- *Not raising the elbow well in the first six inhalation phases*
- *Curving the back while exhaling in the last three phases*
- *Not breathing fully and directly*

Related Warm-Ups for Lotus (see Appendix 1): Butterfly (8), Both Knees to the Side Forward Bend (13), Soles Together Forward Bend (14), Turning and Stretching (15), Hip Opener (28), Soles Together Hip Opener (35)

Related Warm-Ups for Complete Breathing (see Appendix 1): Turning and Stretching (15), Bridge (29), Cat (31), Soles Together Hip Opener (35), Shoulder and Chest Opener (39)

THE FIVE TSIGJONG MOVEMENTS

Loosening the Joints

THE PRELIMINARY PRACTICE of the five Tsigjong movements helps to loosen the various joints, tendons, and nerves of the body. This sequence of movements is a warm-up routine that is part of the original practice of Yantra Yoga. All five movements should be coordinated and synchronized with the breathing and have the same strength and pace. The inhalation and exhalation are direct and complete, yet quick and forceful, through the nose only. Each phase of inhalation and exhalation should be equally strong, complete, and quick, with the same force and same intensity. By inhaling and exhaling quickly and directly and with the strength and energy of the movement, we can very effectively warm up and loosen our joints.

Each of the five Tsigjongs can be linked to the next, creating a continuous flow of energetic movement and breathing. In all Tsigjongs, it is important not to block the breathing after inhaling and not to exhale quicker than inhaling. The individual phases of the Tsigjongs are generally repeated a total of three or five times (five or seven in the case of the last), but if you need to shorten the practice of the Tsigjongs, the movements can be done only one or three times each. Unlike the Lungsangs, which should always be practiced in their entirety, you can choose to do just some of the Tsigjongs rather than all.

11

First Tsigjong | TIGHTENING

I N THE FIRST Tsigjong, Tightening, we contract and relax all five sense organs as well as all the muscles, tendons, and nerves of the body. Specifically, during the exhalation, we contract all the sense organs, tightening the ears, eyes, nose, and the whole body to the point of trembling. Conversely, during the phase of inhalation, we open and relax all tension.

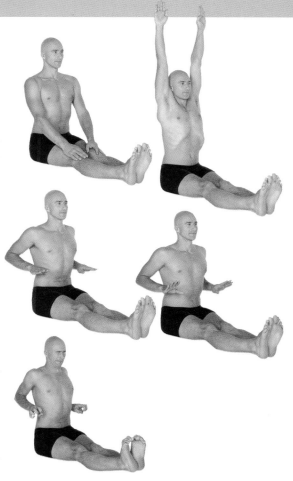

STARTING PHASE
Sit with your legs in front of you, your hands on your knees, and your back straight.

Inhaling directly with strength, raise your arms over your head while expanding your chest.

CENTRAL PHASE
Now exhale, directly and forcefully, bringing your hands to chest level with your elbows back and close to your sides.

Inhaling strongly, let your shoulders and the joints of your hands and feet open while opening your eyes.

Exhaling strongly, tighten, flex, and contract your feet and toes. Pull the root of the tongue down, tighten your eyes shut, and contract all the other sense organs while tensing your whole body to the point of trembling.

Throughout this Tsigjong, keep your back straight and your inhalation and exhalation direct and complete, yet quick and forceful, always through the nose only. Be sure to keep your forearms parallel to the floor. Do not open your elbows to the side or push your feet forward instead of curling your toes.

Now inhale again, relaxing all the tension in your body and opening your eyes, fingers, toes, and shoulders.

Exhale, tightening and tensing your whole body and your sense organs with force and vigor, as before.

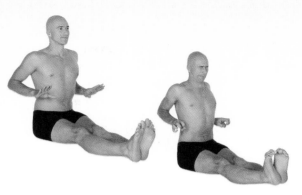

REPETITION
Repeat the alternation of inhaling and exhaling, relaxing and tightening a total of three, five, or seven times in a steady, strong rhythm of breathing and movement.

CONCLUSION
After the final inhalation phase, bring your hands to your knees as you exhale.

Then inhale strongly, stretching your arms upward and fully expanding your chest.

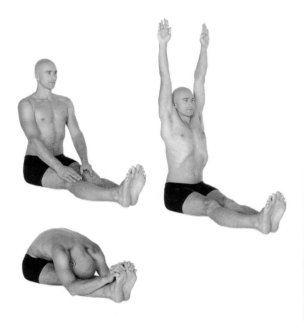

Finally, exhale strongly and bring your fingers to your toes and your forehead to your knees, keeping your back as straight as possible.

This final phase is the same for many of the Yantra Yoga exercises. As you exhale and bend forward, it is important to remember to keep your head in alignment with your spine and your back straight. Bend from the base of your spine rather than from the waist. If you cannot touch your forehead to your knees with your back straight, simply go as far as you are able.

TRANSITION

To link to the next Tsigjong, inhale strongly, raising your arms, and then exhale equally strongly, bringing the soles of your feet together and your hands to your knees.

HEALTH BENEFITS

- *Revitalizes and invigorates the entire organism*
- *Reinforces the condition of the five elements*
- *Improves eyesight and the functioning of the other sense organs*
- *Invigorates the functioning of the pervasive prana, which presides over the movement of the limbs*

Second Tsigjong | SHAKING

T HE SECOND TSIGJONG has three phases: first, we shake only the hands, then the feet, then hands and feet together. To truly benefit from this exercise, it is important to really shake your hands and feet with vigor and intensity.

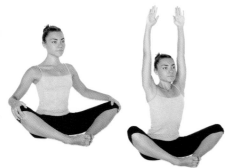

STARTING PHASE

Sit with your back straight, knees wide apart, soles of your feet joined together, and hands on your knees, a position called *tsokyil* in Tibetan.

Inhale with energy, extending your arms up alongside your head.

FIRST PHASE

Quickly exhale with energy and intent, bringing your hands to the level of your armpits, keeping your elbows wide apart. Inhale forcefully, shaking your wrists and fingers vigorously.

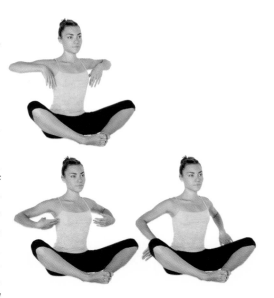

Exhale strongly as you continue to shake your hands and move them downward along the sides of your torso. Inhaling, move your hands back up to the level of your armpits, still shaking them vigorously and with energy. To end, exhale strongly and continue shaking your hands while bringing them down along the sides again.

Put all your energy into the shaking ac-tion so that it is truly vigorous, and con-tinue with the same force as you lower and raise your hands along your sides. Avoid curving your back.

Repeat this sequence three or five times.

Loosening the Joints | The Five Tsigjong Movements

After the last exhalation, inhale energetically, raising your arms up and straightening your legs in front of you.

Then exhale, bringing your fingers to your toes and your forehead to your knees.

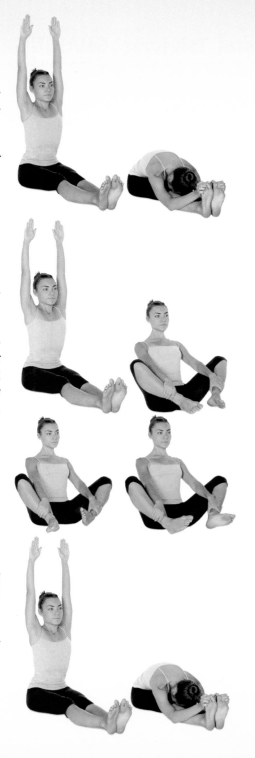

SECOND PHASE

Inhale strongly, raising your arms and expanding your chest.

Exhale quickly, bending your legs and firmly grasping your ankles. Balancing on your buttocks, shake your feet vigorously as you inhale and exhale directly and forcefully for a total of three or five breathing cycles.

After the last phase of exhalation and shaking, inhale quickly and forcefully, raising your arms straight up and parallel and extending your legs in front of you.

Then exhale, bringing your fingers to your toes and your forehead to your knees.

THIRD PHASE

After some practice, once you feel sufficiently confident, you can add the Third Phase to this Tsigjong.

Inhale, raising your arms over your head and fully expanding your chest.

Exhale forcefully while bringing your hands near your armpits, keeping your elbows wide apart. At the same time, lift your feet up and balance on your buttocks with your knees wide apart.

Inhale and exhale as you vigorously shake your wrists, hands, fingers, ankles, and feet. Shake your hands at armpit level during the first inhalation and lower them during the exhalation. Continuing to shake your hands vigorously, bring them back to armpit level as you inhale. Repeat this phase for three or five strong breathing cycles.

CONCLUSION

After the final exhalation, inhale, extending your arms over your head and your legs in front.

Then exhale, bringing your fingers to your toes and your forehead to your knees.

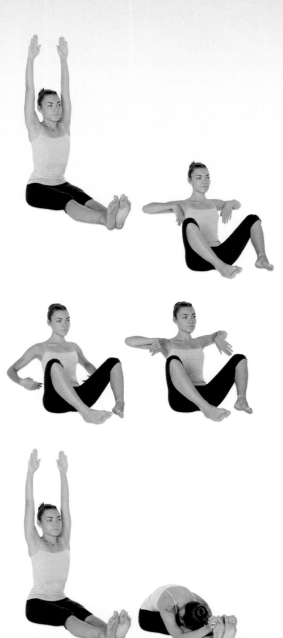

TRANSITION

To link to the next Tsigjong, inhale strongly, raising your arms over your head, then exhale just as strongly, bringing the soles of your feet together and your hands to your knees.

HEALTH BENEFITS

- *Alleviates ailments of all the major and minor ligaments and joints*
- *Improves the condition of the joints and ligaments*

Related Warm-Ups (see Appendix 1): Shaking the Feet (4)

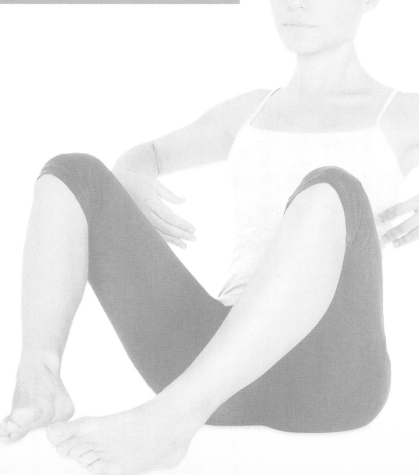

Third Tsigjong │ PULLING

T HE THIRD TSIGJONG, Pulling, has two phases. In the first phase, we focus mostly on loosening the joints of one leg, then the other, with women and men starting on opposite sides. As explained in the Introduction, this is because Yantra Yoga takes subtle energetic differences between females and males into account, a distinction that becomes particularly apparent in the asymmetrical poses. The second phase is done in the same way by both genders, but takes some practice because it involves balancing on the buttocks. In the beginning, you can concentrate on gaining familiarity with the first phase.

STARTING PHASE

Sit with the soles of your feet together, knees wide apart, and hands on your knees.

Inhale forcefully, extending your legs forward and your arms over your head.

FIRST PHASE

Exhaling, grasp the outside of one foot with the corresponding hand and place your other hand on the knee of the same leg.

Women grasp the outside of the right foot with the right hand and place the left hand on the right knee. Men grasp the left foot with the left hand, placing the right hand on the left knee.

If you cannot grasp your foot without bending your knee, just take hold of your ankle.

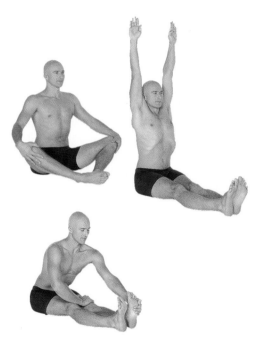

Inhaling energetically, raise your extended leg, keeping your back straight.

Exhaling, bending your leg to bring the sole of your foot to the opposite side above the top of your thigh.

Be sure to bring your foot to your side, beyond the top of your thigh, not just to the groin. Do not push your knees to the floor. Remember to keep your back straight, shoulders open, the straight leg well extended, and your hand on your knee.

Continue by inhaling forcefully, raising your leg diagonally across the extended leg above your knee.

Then exhale forcefully while strongly but smoothly pulling your foot and your knee straight back along the same diagonal direction to the other side, opening the groin well. Repeat the sequence three or five times before switching to the other side.

TRANSITION
To link to the other side, inhale, extending your arms over your head and stretching your leg forward parallel to the other. Then exhale, bringing your fingers to your toes and your forehead to your knees. Return to the beginning of the first phase, inhaling as you raise your arms above your head. Exhale, taking the reverse position with your legs and arms, and repeat the entire first phase sequence three or five times on the opposite side.

In the second round, women grasp the outside of the left foot with the left hand and place the right hand on the left knee. Men grasp the right foot with the right

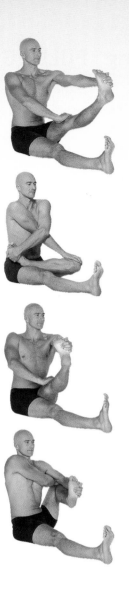

hand, placing the left hand on the right knee.

Conclude by raising your arms while inhaling and bending forward while exhaling, bringing your fingers to your toes and your forehead to your knees.

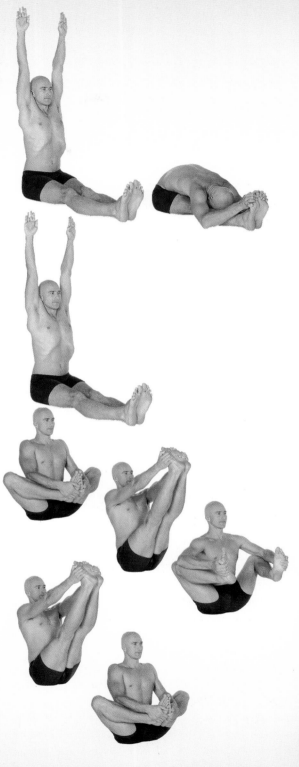

After some practice, once you feel sufficiently confident, you can add the second phase to this Tsigjong. As in the previous phase, all of the inhalations and exhalations are equally deep, vigorous, and brisk.

After the end of the first phase, rise back up as you inhale with strength, extending your arms above your head and keeping your legs extended and your back straight.

Exhale, grasping the outsides of both feet and pulling them together toward your abdomen.

Inhale, extending your legs parallel and straight out at shoulder height.

Exhale, pulling both legs and feet back along your sides, opening your knees.

Inhale, extending your legs parallel and straight out.

Exhale, pulling both feet together toward your navel. Alternate these phases of inhalation and exhalation three or five times.

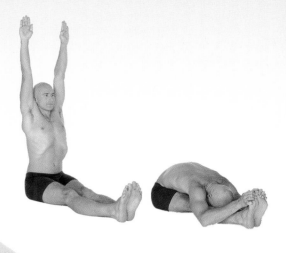

CONCLUSION
Inhale, extending your arms up and your legs forward.

Exhale, bringing your fingers to your toes and your forehead to your knees.

TRANSITION
To link to the next Tsigjong, inhale strongly, open your knees, place the soles of your feet on the floor near your perineum, and extend your arms in front as you pull your-self up onto your knees with your toes curled under and your arms stretched above your head.

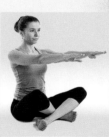

Alternatively, you can come into the kneeling position by crossing your legs close to the pubis and rolling up onto your knees that way. If that is also challenging, simply come to the kneeling position in a way that is comfortable for you.
   Then exhale, sitting on your heels with your hands on your knees.

HEALTH BENEFITS
- *Relieves ailments of the lumbar region*
- *Improves the condition of the major and minor joints*
- *Alleviates disorders of the kidneys*
- *Counteracts problems related to the functioning of the downward-clearing prana, which presides over the ex-cretion of feces and the discharge of urine, semen, and menstrual blood*
- *Tones all functions of the lower body, including reproductive functions*

Related Warm-Ups (see Appendix 1): Rotating the Legs (6)

Fourth Tsigjong | BENDING

THE FOURTH TSIGJONG, Bending, involves twisting and bending the spine and stretching the sides. To enjoy its full benefits, it is particularly important that the spine is well aligned while doing the twisting and bending movements. Throughout this Tsigjong, keep your interlaced fingers directly above your crown, without touching your head, and pull your elbows back as far as possible. As with all of the Tsigjongs, all inhalations and exhalations are equally strong, complete, quick, and dynamic.

STARTING PHASE

Sit on your heels with your hands on your knees, your back straight, and your head aligned with your spine.

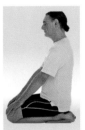

You may need to use some props to make sitting on your heels more comfortable and ensure that your back is correctly aligned. For example, depending on your needs you can place a cushion between your buttocks and your heels or a rolled towel under your ankles.

Inhale forcefully, raising your arms and interlacing your fingers with your palms downward. Keep your hands a few finger-widths above the crown of your head, elbows wide apart and shoulders open.

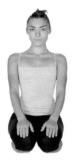

CENTRAL PHASE

Exhaling forcefully, twist your torso to one side, initiating the movement from the root of your spine.

Women start by turning to the right; men start by turning to the left.

Do not push with your elbows and shoulders; let the torsion originate from the root of your spine.

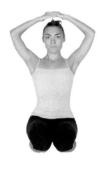

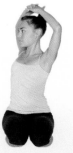

Inhaling with energy, turn back to the center with a smooth yet strong movement.

Exhale and continue the twisting movement to the other side.

Inhale to the center again.

Exhale forcefully while bending to the side from the waist.
  Women start by bending to the right side; men start by bending to the left.

Inhale back to the center.

Without pausing, exhale and bend to the opposite side.

Inhale to the center, then exhale as you twist to the side, as at the beginning.

REPETITION
Repeat the entire sequence of twisting and bending three or five times.
  Remember to keep your inhalations and exhalations direct, strong, and energetic, and do all the movements with equal vigor.

CONCLUSION
After the final inhalation to the center, exhale, stretching your arms forward and bringing your forehead to your knees.

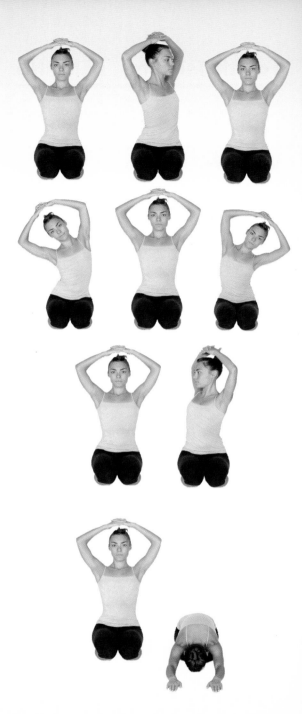

TRANSITION

To link to the next Tsigjong, inhale while rising up on your knees with your arms extended parallel above your head, and roll back to sit on your buttocks. Then exhale, extending your legs forward and bringing your fingers to your toes and your forehead to your knees. Inhale, rising to sitting and placing your hands on your knees, palms up. Rest a moment as you exhale.

HEALTH BENEFITS

- *Relieves and prevents problems of the thoracic and lumbar regions*
- *Alleviates and prevents ailments related to the spine and spinal cord*
- *Benefits the kidneys*
- *Strengthens the tendons of the legs*
- *Reinforces the functioning of the fire-accompanying prana, which presides over the digestive system*

Related Warm-Ups (see Appendix 1): Swinging (1), Transition Training (22)

Fifth Tsigjong | ROTATING

T HE FIFTH TSIGJONG, Rotating, has the unique quality of challenging us to simultaneously engage in both sensory and motor aspects of our awareness as we perform multiple activities at once. It is an excellent exercise for the eyes.

STARTING POSITION
Sit with your legs extended forward one span apart and hands resting on your knees with the palms facing up.

CENTRAL PHASE
Inhaling with energy and intent, join the backs of your hands with the fingers pointing downward, and bring them to the level of your throat by raising your elbows high as you keep your chest open. At the same time as you move your hands upward, turn your feet forward and inward, joining them at the toes.

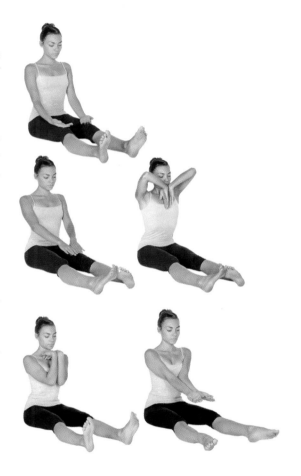

Exhaling, join the elbows at the abdomen in a circular motion without separating your wrists as you lower your hands to the level of your knees with your palms facing upward. At the same time as you move your hands down, turn your feet outward, continuing in an uninterrupted circular motion down and back to center as you inhale and repeat the upward movement with your hands. During the entire process, follow the movement of your right fingers with your right eye, and the movement of your left fingers with your left eye. Repeat the sequence a total of five or seven times.

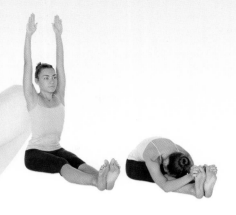

CONCLUSION

Inhale deeply and strongly, energetically extending your arms above your head and expanding your chest.

Exhale, bringing your fingers to your toes and your forehead to your knees.

TRANSITION

If you want to rest at this point, you can lie down and relax with your arms out to the side and your feet slightly apart. Otherwise, continue with the Lungsang movements. If you want to link the fifth Tsigjong directly to the first Lungsang, inhale and raise your arms straight above your head. Exhale, bringing the soles of your feet in front of your perineum and stretching your arms horizontally in front of you to help you rise onto your feet and come into standing with your arms along your sides. If you lay down to relax, roll to one side before coming up into standing.

HEALTH BENEFITS

- *Relieves sensory-motor dysfunctions of the limbs and the head*
- *Alleviates stiffness of the limbs*
- *Improves the condition of the major and minor joints*
- *Counteracts problems related to the pervasive prana*
- *Improves the capacity of harmonious coordination of movements*
- *Strengthens and improves the eyesight*

Related Warm-Ups (see Appendix 1): Shoulder and Chest Opener (39)

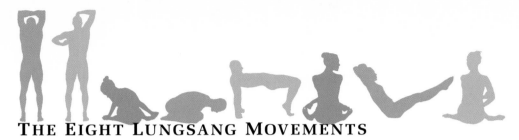

Purifying the Prana

THE PURPOSE OF the eight Lungsangs is to harmonize and strengthen our energies through dynamic and effective exercises that act on the physical level through body movements and on the subtle level through coordination of the breath. Aside from toning and training the body, these movements have the very specific goal of training and developing four different ways of inhaling and exhaling and, especially, four different ways of holding the breath. Performing these movements correctly and with steadfast application progressively improves our awareness and understanding of these modes of breathing. The Lungsangs are the key to harmonizing and reshaping habitual breathing patterns. As a consequence, we can make our body more flexible and fit while improving overall strength and health. Our energy becomes balanced and relaxed, and our vital life force strengthens.

Each of the eight Lungsangs is named after the fundamental aspects of breathing it trains: slow inhalation, open hold, directed hold, quick exhalation, quick inhalation, closed hold, contracted hold, and slow exhalation. Each Lungsang consists of seven phases shaped by a precise rhythm, with the main focus on the central phase of the sequence. Throughout the movements and holds, it is crucial to maintain a correct flow of the rhythm. The timing of each phase is based on either two or four counts, each count corresponding to a heartbeat. Coordinating the inhalations, holds, and exhalations with the count is a fundamental tool for harmonizing the way our breath, and thus our energy, functions. Each of the symmetrical Lungsang movements is repeated three times, while the asymmetrical movements are done only once on each side.

Once you are familiar with the Lungsangs, they can be practiced in a continuous flow where the concluding phase of one merges with the initial phase of the next, without pausing. The Lungsangs are structured in a specific sequence related to the function of the holds, so it is best to practice them in that same order, from the first to the last, without leaving any out. If you do not have much time to dedicate to your practice, you can shorten the session by doing the symmetrical Lungsangs only once.

First Lungsang | INHALING SLOWLY

THE FIRST LUNGSANG trains and develops the experience of long, complete inhalation and open hold. The complete inhalation is achieved by fully and deeply filling the lungs from the bottom up in four counts; the air is then simply retained for two counts without any contracting or blocking. During the open hold, all the muscles and tendons are tensed to the point of slightly trembling, especially the crossed arms and upper part of the body. This tensing of the body actually helps you maintain a relaxed and open hold, without closing or blocking, as you continue to expand and relax the held air.

STARTING PHASE

Stand straight, with your feet and legs parallel and your arms at your sides.

Inhaling in two counts, grasp each arm with the other hand just above the elbow, slightly pressing the inside of each arm with your thumbs. Raise your arms to shoulder height, still within the two-count inhalation.

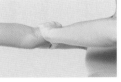 *Women grasp the right arm with the left hand first; men grasp the left arm with the right hand. In this Lungsang, as well as in the fourth and seventh, you do not reverse the position of your hands in the individual phases.*

Exhaling in two counts, lower your arms toward your abdomen while exhaling well from top to bottom.

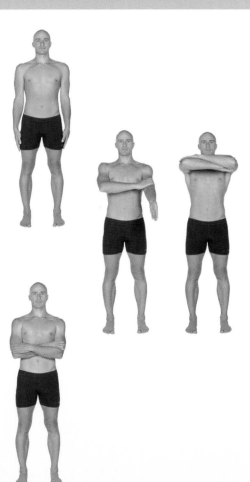

CENTRAL PHASE

In four counts, inhale slowly and fully, starting from the abdomen, as you stretch your arms above your head, expanding the air upward to the chest.

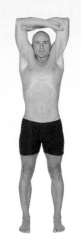

Keep your torso straight to achieve and experience a correct and complete inhalation.

Hold open in this position for two counts, tensing your entire body and vigorously stretching your crossed arms above your head.

Focus the stretch upward, with an outward direction in your elbows, but without letting go of the grip on your arms. Do not push your arms back. Keep your chest open and expanded, with space for more air, as if you wanted to continue to inhale. This will ensure that your hold is not blocked or tensed.

Exhale in two counts, opening your arms wide and lowering them to your sides.

When you exhale, you should not experience any effort or a contraction. If the exhalation is free, simple, and without any tension, your hold is truly open and correct.

CONCLUDING PHASE

Inhale in two counts as you raise your arms straight out to the sides slightly above shoulder height.

Exhaling in two counts, lower your arms back down along your sides.

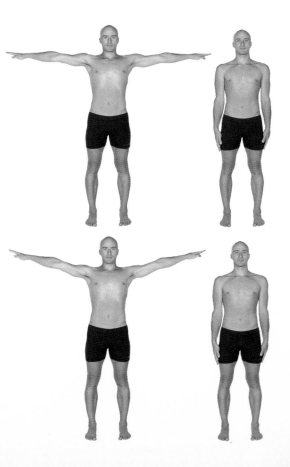

REPETITION

Repeat the entire sequence a total of three times.

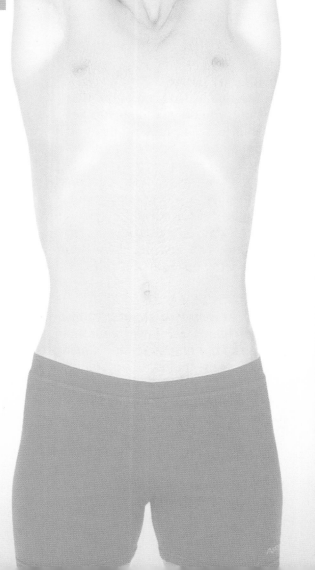

HEALTH BENEFITS

- *Enhances the intellectual faculties*
- *Develops lucidity*
- *Improves the physical condition in general*
- *Relieves ailments related to the five solid organs (heart, lungs, liver, spleen, and kidneys), for instance as a result of having become weakened*

BREATHING CYCLE		COUNTS
Starting Phase	Inhalation	2
	Exhalation	2
Central Phase	Inhalation	**4**
	Open Hold	**2**
	Exhalation	**2**
Concluding Phase	Inhalation	2
	Exhalation	2

Second Lungsang | HOLDING OPEN

T HE SECOND LUNGSANG starts with a deep, full, and complete inhalation, as always from the bottom to the top. The air is then first held open, as in the first Lungsang, and then directed downward while still holding. The position of the arms and elbows in this and the previous Lungsang has the same function as in the Nine Breathings. It helps us open the sides well to allow the breathing to expand. The movement consists of three phases, first on one side, then on the other, and finally on both sides at the same time. Since the first two phases are asymmetrical, women and men start the movement on opposite sides. In the third phase, only the crossing-over movement is reversed for women and men. Each phase is repeated only once.

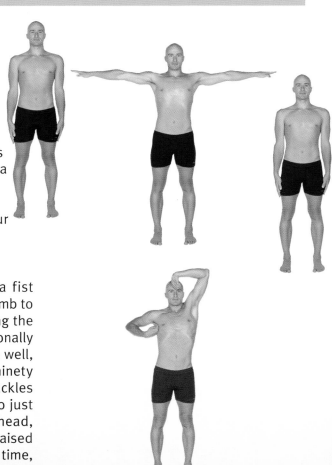

STARTING PHASE
After the final exhalation of the first Lungsang, you are standing straight with your legs and feet parallel and your arms at your sides.

Inhaling in two counts, raise your arms up to the side, reaching out wide at a level slightly above shoulder height.

Exhaling in two counts, lower your arms back to your sides.

FIRST CENTRAL PHASE
Inhaling fully in two counts, form a fist with both hands by bringing your thumb to the base of the ring finger and closing the fingers over the thumb (this is traditionally called a *vajra* fist). Opening your side well,  bring one fist, bent ninety degrees with the knuckles pointing downward, to just in front of your forehead, with the elbow well raised to fully stretch the side. At the same time, press the other fist into your side as you pull it up to your armpit.

In the first phase, women bring the right fist to the forehead while pulling the left fist up to the left armpit; men bring the left fist to the forehead while pulling the right fist up to the right armpit.

Holding open for two counts without constricting or closing the glottis, graze your ear on the same side as your flexed fist as you rotate the fist from your forehead to the nape of your neck.

Continue to hold for another two counts as you complete the rotation of your fist around your head, moving a bit faster to stay in the rhythm and end close to the ear where you started.

During the second two counts of the hold, as you rotate from the nape of your neck to your forehead and to the side, you will notice a subtle shift or directing of the held air as your fist circles around your head. This is what is called directed hold, the main experience of the third Lungsang.

While exhaling in two counts, extend your arms straight out just above shoulder level and lower them to your sides.

FIRST CONCLUDING PHASE

Inhaling in two counts, bring your arms back up to just above shoulder level, spreading them wide apart and opening your chest well.

Exhaling in two counts, lower your arms to your sides.

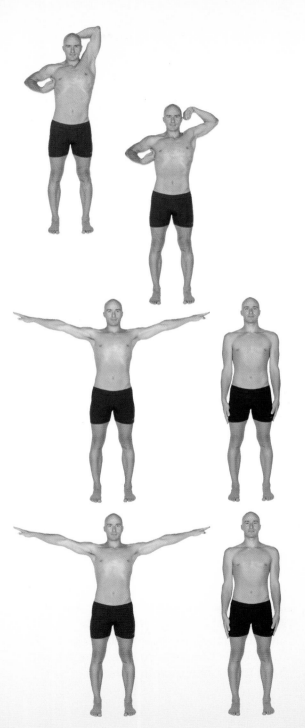

SECOND PHASE

Repeat the entire sequence from the starting position, raising and lowering your arms to your sides once more, then making vajra fists, but this time bringing the opposite fists under the armpit and to your forehead. Then continue with the same sequence of movements as in the first phase, but on the opposite sides.

In the second phase, women bring the left fist to the forehead while pulling the right fist up to the right armpit; men bring the right fist to the forehead while pulling the left fist up to the left armpit.

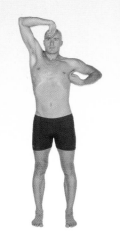

THIRD STARTING PHASE

Start from the standing position that ended the second phase.

Inhaling in two counts, raise your arms up to the side, reaching wide out at a level slightly above shoulder height.

Exhale in two counts as you lower your arms back to your sides.

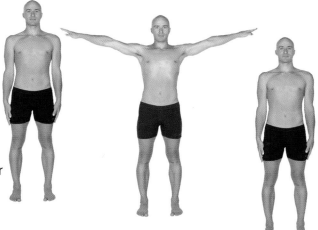

THIRD CENTRAL PHASE

Inhaling in two counts, form vajra fists with both hands, open your arms out to the sides, and raise them up in a circular motion, bringing both fists just in front of your forehead with the knuckles pointing down and the backs of your hands joined as closely as possible. Raise your elbows high to fully expand your sides and chest. Hold a total of four counts, rotating your fists past your ears to cross at the nape of your neck at the end of the first two counts and continuing to circle around your head for the second two counts, ending with both fists close to your ears.

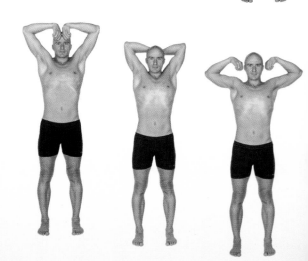

TIBETAN YOGA OF MOVEMENT

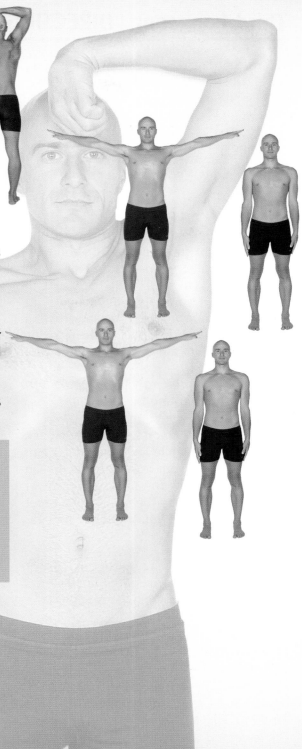

When circling around the head, women pass the right fist over the left as they cross at the nape of the neck; men pass the left fist over the right.

The position and movement of quickly rotating the fists around the head automatically helps the held air to be shifted or directed in the correct way. For the first two counts, the hold is open, and for the second two, it becomes directed.

Exhaling in two counts, extend your arms out and lower them to your sides.

THIRD CONCLUDING PHASE
Inhaling fully in two counts, open your chest well while raising your arms up and extending them wide apart.

Exhaling in two counts, lower your arms back to the sides.

HEALTH BENEFITS
- *Relieves ailments of the thoracic region*
- *Eases problems with the arms and shoulders*
- *Alleviates neurological disorders*
- *Improves the functioning of the small and large joints of the limbs*

BREATHING CYCLE		COUNTS
Starting Phase	Inhalation	2
	Exhalation	2
Central Phase	Inhalation	**2**
	Open Hold	**2**
	Directed Hold	**2**
	Exhalation	**2**
Concluding Phase	Inhalation	2
	Exhalation	2

Third Lungsang | DIRECTING

THE THIRD OF the eight Lungsangs focuses on directed hold. This Lungsang gives you a much deeper experience of directed hold than the subtle directed hold that occurs in the previous movement. Aside from training you in directed hold, this movement also teaches you how you enter into directed hold from open hold, so it helps you develop smooth breathing and holding. This Lungsang is done one time on each side. Women and men start on opposite sides.

STARTING PHASE

After the final exhalation of the second Lungsang, you are standing with your feet and legs parallel, arms to your sides.

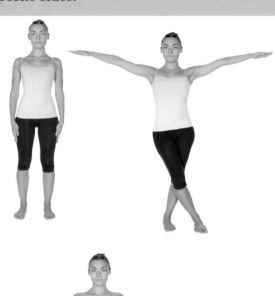

Inhale in two counts while raising your arms up and open to the sides and crossing one leg over the other, placing the crossing foot on the floor along the outside of the standing foot.
   Women cross the right leg over the left; men cross the left leg over the right.

Exhaling in two counts, slide your back foot to the side while lowering yourself to the floor so that your front knee is crossed over the other. At the same time, lower your arms and grasp the soles of your feet so that the flats of your thumbs join your big toes.

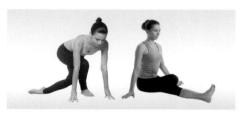

   If necessary, you can help yourself down by placing your hands on the floor for balance. If the sitting position is difficult, try crossing your legs more loosely or extend the lower leg out in front.

CENTRAL PHASE

Keeping your back straight and your knees crossed over each other, inhale in two counts, extending your torso upward as you turn slightly to the open side (the side with the leg on the bottom). As you inhale, start filling from the abdomen and expand into the chest.

Do not turn your neck when you twist to the side; keep it in line with the center of your torso.

Holding open and keeping your torso extended, twist toward the other side. Start the twisting movement from the root of the spine and gradually turn your whole spine, twisting as far to the side as possible in a total of two counts.

Continuing to hold for two more counts, bend over your upper thigh, keeping your back as straight as possible. In this way, the held air is automatically directed to the side and you clearly experience directed hold.

Exhale in two counts while continuing to stretch your torso over your thigh, bringing your forehead as close to the floor as possible.

CONCLUDING PHASE

Inhaling fully in two counts, extend your arms over your head, keeping them straight and parallel as you fully open your chest, and straighten your legs to the front.

Exhaling smoothly in two counts, bring your fingers to your toes and your forehead to your knees.

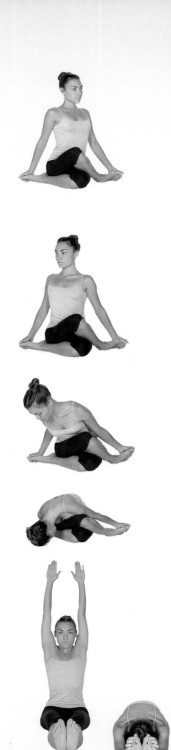

REPETITION

Repeat the sequence on the opposite side, inhaling in two counts as you rise back up and open your arms wide to the sides, keeping your legs stretched out in front of you. Exhaling in two counts, cross your legs the opposite way and continue the sequence of movements on this side as you did before on the previous side.

In the second round, women cross the left leg over the right and men cross the right leg over the left to come into the knee-over-knee sitting position as before.

HEALTH BENEFITS

- *Relieves conditions caused by the weakening or malfunction of the five solid organs (heart, lungs, liver, spleen, and kidneys) and six hollow organs (stomach, small intestine, large intestine, gall bladder, urinary bladder, and seminal vesicles or ovaries)*
- *Alleviates problems related to the lumbar region and waist area as well as the spine and spinal cord*
- *Eases pain in the rib cage*
- *Counteracts problems caused by the fire-accompanying prana, such as poor digestion*

Related Warm-Ups (see Appendix 1): Swinging (1), Crossed Knee Stretch (17), Knee over Knee (18), Supine Twist (27)

BREATHING CYCLE		COUNTS
Starting Phase	Inhalation	2
	Exhalation	2
Central Phase	Inhalation	**2**
	Open Hold	**2**
	Directed Hold	**2**
	Exhalation	**2**
Concluding Phase	Inhalation	2
	Exhalation	2

Fourth Lungsang | EXHALING QUICKLY

THE FOURTH LUNGSANG is for training and experiencing quick exhalation. As in the first Lungsang, here again we train the slow inhalation, followed by an open hold before the main focus of this exercise, where we press the arms to the abdomen to facilitate a quick but complete exhalation.

STARTING PHASE

Until you are familiar with practicing the eight Lungsangs in an uninterrupted succession, you can start this sequence sitting with your legs extended and your hands on your knees.

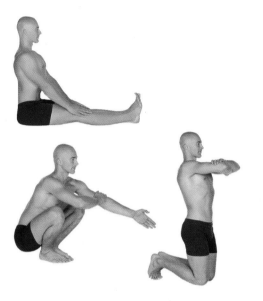

From the concluding phase of the previous Lungsang, inhale in two counts as you rise up to sitting, plant the soles of your feet near your trunk, and roll forward to come up onto your knees with your toes curled under while crossing your arms and bringing them to shoulder level.

Cross your arms in the same way as in the first Lungsang. Women grasp the right arm above the elbow with the left hand first; men grasp the left arm with the right hand. The position of the arms is not reversed in subsequent rounds.

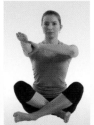

As in the transition to the fourth Tsigjong, if it is difficult to come up in this way, you can cross your legs and roll forward and up onto your knees. If that is also challenging, simply come to the kneeling position in a way that is comfortable for you.

Exhale smoothly in two counts, pressing the tops of your feet to the floor and lowering your crossed arms to beneath your rib cage while bending forward with your back straight.

CENTRAL PHASE

Inhale fully in four counts, filling from the bottom up and straightening your spine as you come up onto your knees. Leave the tops of your feet flat on the floor while you raise your arms, still crossed over each other, to shoulder level.

Holding open and relaxed for two counts, lower your crossed arms to the area below your rib cage while keeping your chest open.

In two counts, exhale quickly and forcefully from your nostrils while pushing your crossed arms toward your navel and bending forward with your back straight as you bring your forehead to the floor.

This sequence is the main focus of the fourth Lungsang. To have the right experience of quick exhalation, it is crucial that you keep your back straight and your buttocks resting on your heels as you bend forward, even if you cannot touch the floor with your forehead. Do not lift your buttocks off your heels or bend your neck.

CONCLUDING PHASE

Inhaling in two counts, come up onto your knees with your toes curled under as you extend your arms over your head and expand your chest.

Exhaling in two counts, sit back on your heels with your arms at your sides and the tops of your feet flat on the floor.

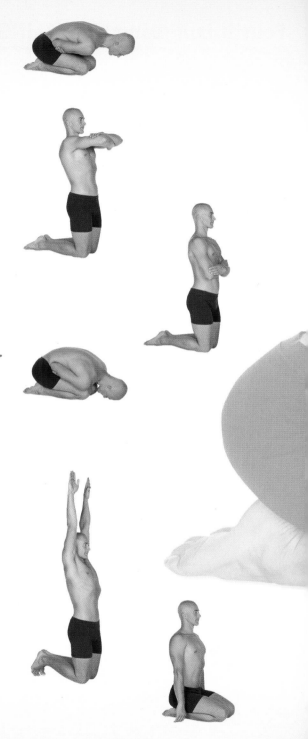

REPETITION

To complete the fourth Lungsang, repeat the entire sequence two more times, except that you start from the kneeling position with your arms along your sides. In the second and third repetitions, inhale in two counts, cross your arms in the same way as in the first round, and come up onto your knees with your toes curled under. Then continue the sequence as before, from the long inhalation, open hold, fast exhalation, and final inhalation until you exhale and sit back on your heels.

HEALTH BENEFITS

- *Invigorates the five solid and six hollow organs*
- *Alleviates problems caused by malfunctioning of the five solid and six hollow organs*
- *Relieves ailments of the tendons, ligaments, and major and minor joints*
- *Harmonizes wind energy imbalances manifesting in the areas governed by the pervasive and the downward-clearing pranas*

Related Warm-Up (see Appendix 1): Transition Training (22)

Breathing Cycle		Counts
Starting Phase	Inhalation	2
	Exhalation	2
Central Phase	Inhalation	**4**
	Open Hold	**2**
	Exhalation	**2**
Concluding Phase	Inhalation	2
	Exhalation	2

Fifth Lungsang | INHALING QUICKLY

THE FIFTH LUNGSANG is for training in inhaling quickly and directly. It also introduces us to the experience of closed hold, the main focus of the sixth Lungsang. During the closed hold, the held air is blocked and locked downward and the sides are tightened so that the hold is felt below the navel. The dynamics of the breathing and movement facilitate that experience.

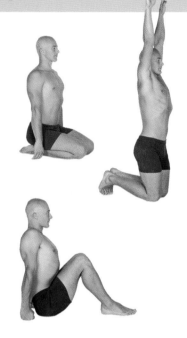

STARTING PHASE

Continue from the last position of the previous Lungsang, seated on your heels with your arms at your sides.

Inhale in two counts and extend your arms over your head while curling your toes under and coming up on your knees.

Exhaling in two counts, roll back to sit on your buttocks with your knees close together near your chest and your hands in vajra fists along your sides.

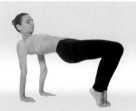

If it is difficult to use the vajra fist, you can make a normal fist with your thumbs on the outside, or you can simply place your palms on the floor by your sides. Also, you may find that you need to place your hands slightly farther back to feel more stable and comfortable.

CENTRAL PHASE

Inhale quickly in two counts while raising your pelvis up, bringing your torso parallel to the floor and supporting your weight on your fists and toes. Hold closed in this position for two counts while tensing your whole body.

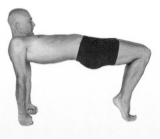

Keep your knees together or at least parallel. Also, for the experience of closed hold, it is paramount to keep your chin tucked in and not throw your head back. The air is blocked below the navel, and your abdominal muscles and sides are tightened. You should feel the pressure of the hold blocked below the navel.

Now exhale slowly and fully for four counts as you gradually lower your buttocks back to the floor, bringing your chest to your thighs and the underside of your chin to rest on your knees.

If you cannot rest your chin on your knees, bring it above your knees or as far as your capacity allows. Try to keep your shoulders open.

CONCLUDING PHASE
Inhale in two counts, extending your arms over your head and expanding your chest as you stretch your legs in front of you.

Exhale in two counts, bringing your forehead to your knees and your fingers to your toes.

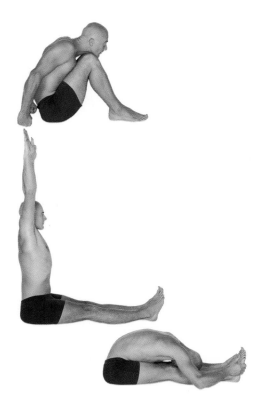

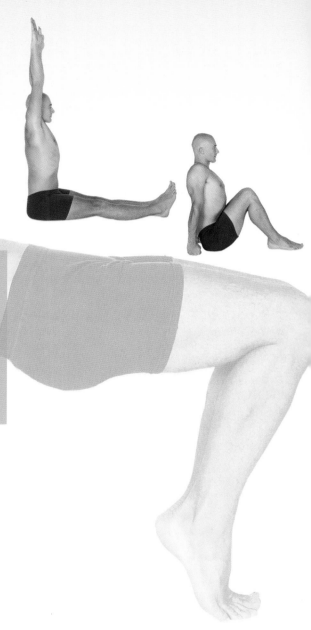

REPETITION

Repeat the entire sequence two more times, starting by inhaling as you rise back up, and extend your arms over your head.

Exhaling in two counts, bring your knees to your chest, and place your hands in vajra fists along your sides. Then continue as before, inhaling quickly, holding closed, exhaling slowly, inhaling, and exhaling. Repeat one last time to end after the third concluding phase.

HEALTH BENEFITS

- *Strengthens the spine and spinal cord*
- *Invigorates the lungs and heart*
- *Improves the condition of the major and minor joints*
- *Alleviates problems related to the ascending prana, which presides over the faculties of speech and breathing, as well as the pervasive prana*

Breathing Cycle		Counts
Starting Phase	Inhalation	2
	Exhalation	2
Central Phase	Inhalation	**2**
	Closed Hold	**2**
	Exhalation	**4**
Concluding Phase	Inhalation	2
	Exhalation	2

Sixth Lungsang | HOLDING CLOSED

THE SIXTH LUNGSANG is for training and experiencing closed hold. The seven phases of the movement serve as a precise guide for entering into closed hold without forcing and for closing the hold at the right time to ensure a correct application.

It is important to remember that the purpose of all eight Lungsangs is to retrain and reshape our breathing patterns and habitual ways of breathing. In this way, they effectively create the conditions that guide the breath safely through the different movements and holds. With this in mind, the breathing needs to be fluid and smooth throughout the sequences of movement to avoid inadvertent "microholds" as a consequence of forcing or tensing the breathing. We only hold when the precise condition is created by the previous phases of breathing and movement. This sixth Lungsang is an especially good example of the application of this principle. In this case, to correctly experience closed hold, the position will guide our breath to fill mainly the lower part of the lungs. As a result, the hold is experienced in the lower abdominal area, with only a little breath in the upper chest.

Physically, this is achieved by crossing your arms firmly over your upper chest while inhaling and straightening your back. In this position, with the chest squeezed by the crossed arms, the inhaled air is unable to expand into the upper chest and is thus guided to expand into the area of the lower lungs. The posture itself creates the ideal conditions for accurately training and experiencing closed hold. After the inhalation, the air is held and the head is rotated and lowered, moving what little breath is in the chest down toward the abdomen. When the chin is finally closed at the chest, the closed hold is clearly experienced. With your chin on the chest, the air is blocked below your navel and controlled by the tightened sides and the straight spine. Continuing to rotate your head adds the experience of directed hold.

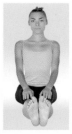

STARTING PHASE
Until you are familiar with practicing the eight Lungsangs in an uninterrupted succession, you can start this sequence sitting with your legs extended and your hands on your knees.

Inhaling in two counts, rise back up from the final exhalation of the previous Lungsang, spreading your arms and legs wide apart and opening your chest well at the same time.

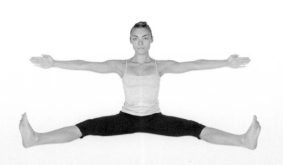

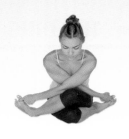

Exhaling in two counts, cross your legs, knee over knee, with your feet pointing backward. At the same time, cross your arms high on your chest, with your upper arm on the same side as your upper leg, bringing your hands to your feet and joining your thumbs with your big toes.

In the first round, women cross the left arm and left leg on top; men cross the right arm and right leg on top.

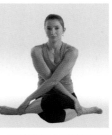

If some aspects of this position are difficult for you, a number of modifications are possible. If you cannot grab hold of your toes or even your feet, you can either grab your ankles or even your knees or thighs. What is important is to have your arms crossed high over your chest so that you can experience how the inhaled air is automatically directed down toward the abdomen by the joint dynamic of the movement and position. If you cannot cross both legs, leave the bottom leg straight, in which case a thin cushion or firm

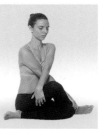

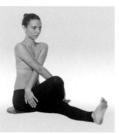

prop under your buttocks can help ensure the proper alignment of your spine.

You may need to help your legs into position with your hands.

CENTRAL PHASE
Inhaling in two counts, straighten your torso and arch your head and neck back.

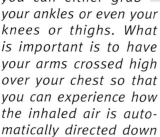

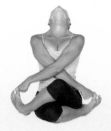

It is important to arch your head as far back as possible so that your spine is thoroughly straightened. Additionally, to experience the correct characteristic of the in-halation, it is crucial to keep your upper chest closed even if you are only able to reach your shins or thighs with your hands.

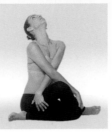

Holding closed for two counts, rotate your head toward the open side, graze your shoulder on that side with your ear, and continue by rolling your head to the center of your body, pushing your chin down as you keep your sides tightened and your spine as straight as possible.

In this first part of the movement, women start the rotation of the head on the right side and men on the left side.

Apply directed hold for two more counts as you stretch your chin over your other shoulder, with your head vertical and your back straight.

Exhaling in two counts, uncross your arms and bring your hands to the floor by your sides as you turn your head to face forward, keeping your back straight.

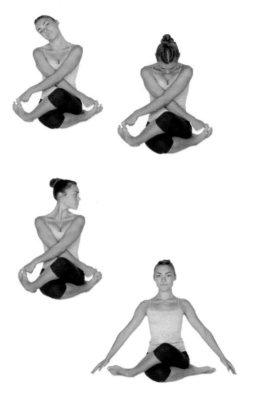

CONCLUDING PHASE

Inhaling in two counts, raise your arms over your head and extend your legs forward.

Exhaling in two counts, bring your fingers to your toes and your forehead to your knees.

REPETITION

Repeat the sequence on the opposite side, inhaling in two counts as you raise your torso up and open your arms and legs wide to the sides. Exhaling in two counts, cross your arms and legs the opposite way and continue the sequence with the reverse movements.

In the second round, women cross the right arm and right leg on top and start the rotation of the head on the left side. Men cross the left arm and left leg on top and start the rotation of the head on the right side.

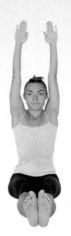

HEALTH BENEFITS

- *Relieves nerve damage affecting and impairing the five sense organs as well as related ailments of the brain*
- *Alleviates and prevents conditions related to the ascending prana and the life-sustaining prana, including anxiety, agitation, and depression*
- *Sharpens the intellect and memory*

Related Warm-Ups (see Appendix 1): Crossed Knee Stretch (17), Knee over Knee (18), Supine Twist (27), Neck Roll (37)

BREATHING CYCLE		COUNTS
Starting Phase	Inhalation	2
	Exhalation	2
Central Phase	Inhalation	**2**
	Closed Hold	**2**
	Directed Hold	**2**
	Exhalation	**2**
Concluding Phase	Inhalation	2
	Exhalation	2

Seventh Lungsang | CONTRACTING

T HE SEVENTH LUNGSANG is for training and developing contracted hold, which is characterized by a backward pull of the abdomen toward the spine. The dynamics of the movement, breathing, and holding facilitate this experience and lock of the hold below the navel and of the navel being drawn back toward the spine.

This Lungsang is not advised for people with serious pathologies of the lower back. If you have this kind of challenge, it is better to apply the simpler version described below or to avoid this exercise until you feel fit enough to perform it without any risk.

STARTING PHASE

Until you are familiar with practicing the eight Lungsangs in an uninterrupted succession, you can start this sequence from a sitting position with your legs stretched in front of you and your hands on your knees.

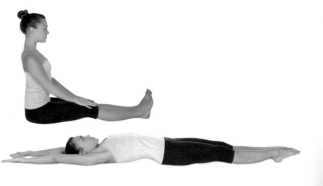

Coming up from the final exhalation of the sixth Lungsang, inhale in two counts, extending your arms over your head, and roll back on your spine, vigorously stretching your arms over your head and pointing your toes as you tense your whole body.

Exhaling in two counts, extend your arms down along your sides with your palms on the floor.

CENTRAL PHASE

Inhale forcefully and quickly in two counts while crossing your arms over your head and further tensing your legs with your toes pointed.

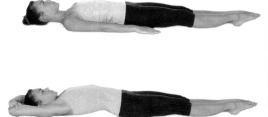

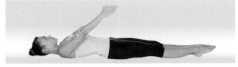

Cross your arms in the same way as in the first Lungsang. Women grasp the right arm with the left hand first, and men grasp the left arm with the right hand. The position of the arms is not reversed in subsequent rounds.

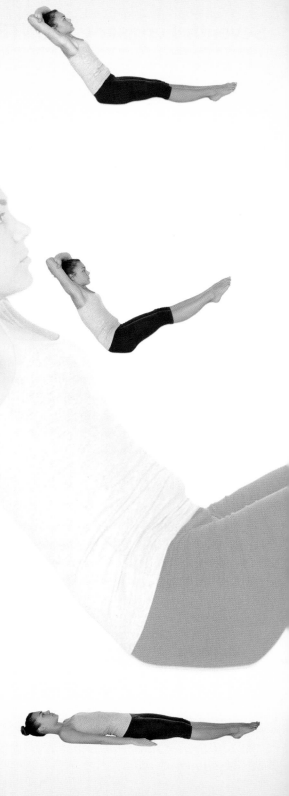

Holding open for two counts, raise your torso to a backward inclined position, keeping your crossed arms well stretched above your head.

Come up onto your sitting bones, keeping your back as straight as possible. Doing the movement correctly automatically gives you control of your abdominal muscles and creates the correct conditions for contracted hold. If you have difficulty coming up into the correct position, you can first come up with your crossed arms in front and then bring them over your head and back. Lift your torso to your capacity.

Holding contracted for another two counts, lift your extended legs off the floor.

Lifting the legs adds firm backward control of the abdominal muscles for a full experience of the characteristics of contracted hold. The position is correct when you remain stable and balanced on your buttocks without raising your legs and torso too much. Ideally, your body should form an obtuse angle.

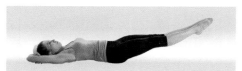

For the modified version of this Lungsang, leave your torso on the floor and just lift your legs a little, keeping your legs and crossed arms tense and controlled. The main point is to feel the tightness and backward pulling of your abdominal muscles. Regardless of whether you raise your upper body, you will still be able to experience the main characteristic of the contracted hold.

Exhale in two counts, lying back with your arms relaxed along your sides.

CONCLUDING PHASE

Inhaling in two counts, extend your arms over your head as you fully expand your chest.

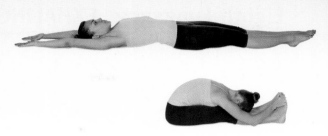

Exhaling in two counts, come up to bring your forehead to your knees and your fingers to your toes.

As always, it is important to have your back correctly aligned and release the tension in the lower back while bending forward without blocking or tensing your breathing or the movement.

REPETITION

Repeat the entire sequence two more times, inhaling as you raise your torso up and roll onto your back with your arms extended over your head. Then continue as before, concluding by exhaling and bringing your forehead to your knees and your fingers to your toes.

HEALTH BENEFITS
- *Alleviates ailments of the spine and spinal cord*
- *Relieves disorders of the six hollow organs*
- *Counteracts problems related to the fire-accompanying prana, such as poor digestion*
- *Benefits digestion in general*

Breathing Cycle		Counts
Starting Phase	Inhalation	2
	Exhalation	2
Central Phase	Inhalation	2
	Open Hold	2
	Contracted Hold	2
	Exhalation	2
Concluding Phase	Inhalation	2
	Exhalation	2

Eighth Lungsang | EXHALING SLOWLY

T HE LAST OF the eight Lungsangs focuses on the experience of a slow and smooth full exhalation. Correct exhalation, emptying fully and evenly from top to bottom, is essential for the harmonious flow of our breathing. It is a crucial factor in strengthening, relaxing, and balancing our vital energy.

STARTING PHASE

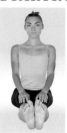

Until you are familiar with practicing the eight Lungsangs in an uninterrupted succession, you can start this sequence from a sitting position with your legs stretched in front of you and your hands on your knees.

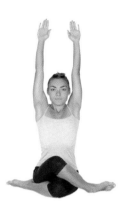

Inhaling fully in two counts, rise back up from the final exhalation of the previous Lungsang, crossing your legs knee over knee with your feet pointing backward while extending your arms over your head and opening your chest. Both buttocks are on the floor.

In the first round, women cross the right leg over the left, men the left leg over the right.

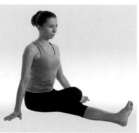

If this position is difficult for you, try crossing your legs more loosely or extending your lower leg out in front. If necessary, first help yourself into the crossed-leg position and then inhale, raising your arms above the head.

Exhaling in two counts, extend your arms along your sides while bending forward a little with your back straight and your head aligned.

CENTRAL PHASE

Inhaling in two counts, reach from behind and grab your arm on the open side just above the elbow and form a vajra fist. While straightening your back, rotate and open your shoulders to fully expand the air in your chest.

In the first round, women grab the left arm with the right hand and men grab the right arm with the left hand.

It is crucial to breathe deeply in this phase, expanding and opening your chest well. If you cannot grab hold of your arm, simply reach behind as far as you can while keeping your back straight.

Applying directed hold for two counts, bring your vajra fist below your navel with a controlled movement to direct the air downward.

Do this movement with strength and intent.

Exhaling slowly and completely in four counts, turn toward your upper thigh with your back straight and bend forward to bring your forehead as close to the floor as possible.

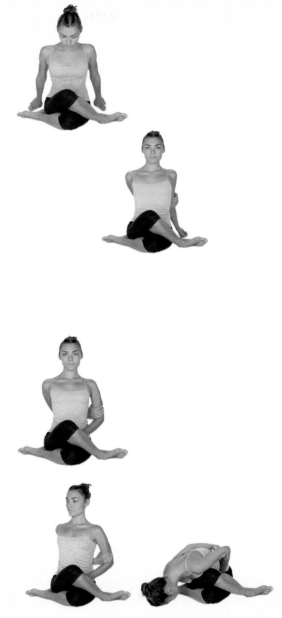

CONCLUDING PHASE

Inhaling from bottom to top in two counts and fully expanding your chest, release your arms and raise them over your head as you bring your legs forward.

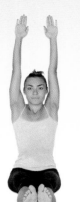

Exhaling in two counts, bend forward from the base of your spine to bring your forehead to your knees and your fingers to your toes.

REPETITION

Repeat the entire sequence on the other side, inhaling in two counts as you rise back up and cross your legs, knee over knee, with your feet pointing backward.

In the second round, women cross the left leg over the right and men cross the right leg over the left. Women grab the right arm with the left hand and men grab the left arm with the right hand.

TRANSITION

As at the end of the Tsigjong group, if you want to rest at this point, you can lie down and relax with your arms out to the side and your feet slightly apart. Otherwise, continue with the Tsadul group.

HEALTH BENEFITS

- *Balances and harmonizes the functions of the five elements*
- *Strengthens the solid and hollow organs*
- *Alleviates problems related to malfunctioning of the solid and hollow organs*
- *Relieves disorders related to the fire-accompanying and downward-clearing pranas*
- *Aids the processes of digestion and elimination*

Related Warm-Ups (see Appendix 1): Swinging (1), Crossed Knee Stretch (17), Knee over Knee (18), Supine Twist (27)

BREATHING CYCLE		COUNTS
Starting Phase	Inhalation	2
	Exhalation	2
Central Phase	Inhalation	**2**
	Directed Hold	**2**
	Exhalation	**4**
Concluding Phase	Inhalation	2
	Exhalation	2

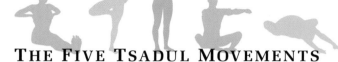

THE FIVE TSADUL MOVEMENTS
Controlling the Energy Channels

THE CHARACTERISTIC FUNCTION of the Tsadul movements is to help soften the muscles while opening and controlling the physical and energetic channels. The Tibetan word *tsa* refers to the channels that run throughout the body, including both physical channels like nerves, veins, and arteries as well as subtle and immaterial *nadis* or energy channels. *Dul* is to control, coordinate, or conquer; in the context of practice it means to optimize and make as efficient and functional as possible. This series of exercises, along with the related pranayama breathing exercise, reactivates the correct circulation of prana within our channels and eliminates all the defects hindering this extremely important function of our life energy.

It is best to start this group with the Tsadul pranayama, a highly effective method for equalizing the smooth and rough aspects of our breathing and balancing our solar and lunar energies. This pranayama creates the ideal conditions to allow the five Tsadul movement sequences to harmonize our subtle energies. Each Tsadul exercise starts with a slow and direct inhalation that leads into a central phase, where we maintain a condition of open hold. We end with a forceful exhalation of all the stale air through the mouth, emitting an aspirated "HA" sound. The inhalations and exhalations do not follow a specific count, but the inhalations are ideally at least four counts, and the

57

quality of the exhalations is sudden and forceful. As with all Yantra Yoga exercises, the movements and breathing are always coordinated with each other. Perform these movements with harmonious strength and presence, with intent, but at the same time never strain or force your body beyond its limits. When performed correctly, the movements themselves help us overcome our limits with training and steadfast, constant application.

Each Tsadul can be done three, five, seven, or more times according to your capacity and ability to hold your breath in an open and controlled way. If you feel any discomfort in holding your breath, until you are more familiar with these sequences it might be easier and more comfortable to perform the exercises without holding, coordinating the movements with the inhalation and exhalation, more like warm-up exercises. The first, third, and fifth Tsaduls are especially suited for this approach. Each of the Tsadul movement sequences is generally repeated three times. If you have limited time, you can shorten this group of movements by doing each only once. The second Tsadul, being symmetrical, is done three times on each side, or only once on each side in the short version of the practice.

Tsadul Breathing | BALANCING SOLAR AND LUNAR ENERGY

T HE MAIN AIM of this exercise is to balance the forces of the solar and lunar energy. To obtain this equilibrium, you inhale through the nostril linked to the solar energy channel and exhale through the nostril linked to the lunar energy channel. In this pranayama, the inhalations are smooth and direct and the exhalations are rough and indirect. Inhaling on the solar side has the effect of strengthening the solar energy and neutralizing the agitation that can be caused by an excess of energy on the lunar side.

Beyond having a warm-up effect, this pranayama allows us to work at the level of our energies. As a consequence, it helps our thoughts settle and encourages the positive aspects of balanced and strong energy to manifest. It also creates the perfect conditions for subsequently performing the five Tsadul exercises.

THE PRANAYAMA
Sit in Vairochana pose or in any of the modified sitting positions suggested in the chapter on the Nine Purification Breathings, above. After relaxing with two or three complete, direct, and slow inhalations and exhalations, close one nostril with your ring finger and exhale the air forcefully and indirectly through the opposite nostril, applying what is called rough indirect breathing.

Women close the right nostril with the left ring finger and exhale from the left nostril; men close the left nostril with the right ring finger and exhale from the right nostril.

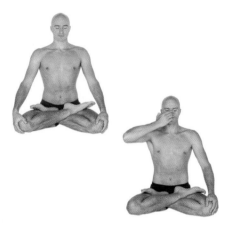

INDIRECT BREATHING

In indirect breathing, you should feel that the air is controlled at the glottis or back of your throat and hear a rasping sound. For an easy demonstration of direct and indirect exhalation, hold a piece of paper under your nose and exhale onto it, first directly, then indirectly. A direct exhalation will make the paper move, while the indirect method will not.

Then close the opposite nostril with your thumb, open the other by lifting your ring finger, and inhale through the open nostril, drawing the air in calmly and smoothly with a long and direct breath. After repeating this phase three, seven, or more times, the force of the breath will shift and be stronger through the solar nostril.

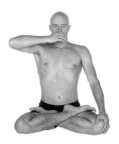

To check the strength of the air, put the back of your hand under your nostrils and exhale onto it. After the exercise, the air should emerge more strongly from the solar nostril or with equal force from both nostrils. The flow of air from the lunar nostril should diminish. In order for this to happen, it is crucial that the exhalation is truly indirect and faster than the inhalation.

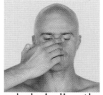
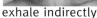

exhale indirectly

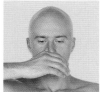

inhale directly

Once the smooth and rough aspects of the breath are equalized and the strength of the solar and lunar sides is balanced, inhale calmly and smoothly through the solar nostril and hold this neutral air for as long as is comfortable, applying an open, relaxed hold and allowing the air to pervade the entire body. Then exhale indirectly as before. Repeat three, five, or more times.

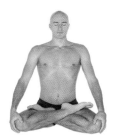

Maintaining full control of your exhalation after the hold will enable you to repeat the process several times without effort. If at any point you feel any discomfort or that you have been forcing yourself to stay too long in the hold, change air by inhaling and exhaling one or three times as in the last three exhalations of the Nine Purification Breathings.

First Tsadul | MASSAGING

THE FIRST TSADUL includes a vigorous massage from the chest to the toes that helps us relax muscular tension and open the energy channels.

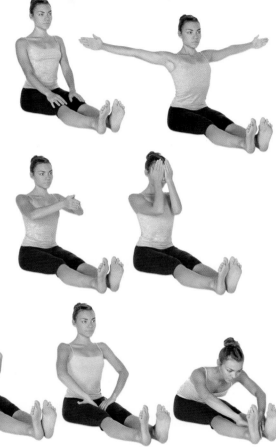

STARTING PHASE
Sit with your back straight, legs extended in front, and hands resting on your knees.

Inhale slowly and directly, fully expanding your chest and opening your arms wide apart to the sides.

CENTRAL PHASE
Holding open, slap your hands together with force and rub your palms together energetically to create some heat. Then gently press the palms over your eyes and let the heat be transferred to them.

Still holding open, massage both sides of your body energetically, pulling your hands firmly from your face along your torso and especially the inside of your legs to your toes, with your fingers facing inward and your thumbs facing outward.

When you reach your toes, turn your hands around and, with your fingers turned outward and your thumbs inward, massage from your ankles back up along your legs, this time focusing on the outside of your legs,

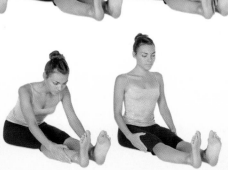

continuing up the sides of the torso all the way to your armpits, bringing your thumbs under your armpits and your fingertips to the base of your neck. Still holding open, energetically repeat the process of massaging your body by pressing and pulling your hands up and down your sides and legs three, five, seven, or more times, according to your capacity to hold your breath.

If you like, when you do this Tsadul, you can apply oil to your body and vigorously rub it into your skin. As an alternative to oil, which increases blood flow and has a warming effect, you can also use rubbing alcohol, which causes blood vessels to constrict and hence decreases fluid accumulation and inflammation. Both relax the muscles and help open the energy channels.

When you reach your capacity to hold your breath, vigorously extend your arms and legs apart and exhale the stale air from your mouth, forcefully emitting an aspirated "HA" sound.

Let the fierce exhalation with "HA" be the driving force of the strong movement, bringing your hands from your neck straight out above your open legs. Emit the "HA" without using your vocal cords or attempting to pronounce it, fully expelling the remaining air from your lungs with your mouth open.

If you find it difficult at the beginning to do the movements while holding your breath, you can perform this exercise without the hold, simply coordinating the movements with your inhalation and exhalation. In that case, exhale while massaging downward and inhale while massaging upward.

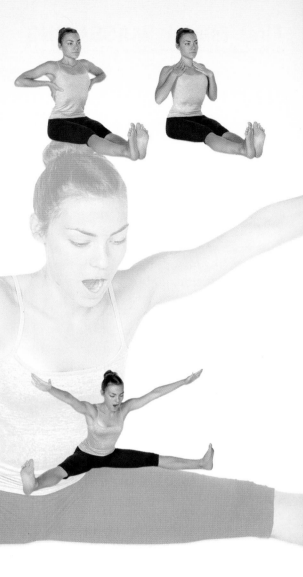

REPETITION

Inhale, bringing your legs together and your hands on your knees. Exhale, remaining in the position.

Repeat the entire sequence two more times, starting by inhaling fully as you open your arms wide.

CONCLUDING PHASE

If you want to conclude this Tsadul or repeat the entire sequence, after emitting the "HA" on exhaling, keep your legs open wide as you inhale and exhale forcefully and quickly three times, raising your arms up on the inhalation and bringing your fingers to your toes and your forehead to or toward the floor on the exhalation. Repeat this process of inhaling quickly and bending forward to reach your toes as you exhale a total of three times.

TRANSITION

To link to the next Tsadul, inhale, bringing the soles of your feet near your perineum while moving your arms in front and up, and stand up with your arms parallel above your head. Exhale, bringing your arms along your sides, standing with your legs and feet parallel.

When standing up, it is important not to hold or block your breathing but to keep inhaling long and direct.

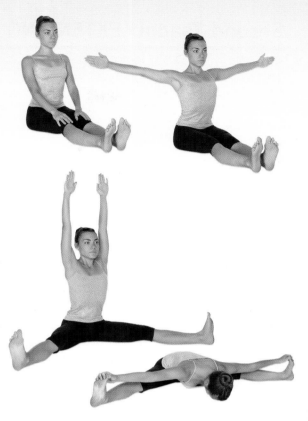

HEALTH BENEFITS

- *Alleviates disorders of lymphatic circulation and the skin*
- *Harmonizes imbalances of wind energy*
- *Counteracts problems caused by the impaired or weakened functioning of the pervasive prana*
- *Relieves eye strain and benefits eyesight in general*

Second Tsadul | EXTENDING THE ANKLES

T HE SECOND TSADUL, trains balance and works with the lower body and downward-clearing prana. You may need to get accustomed to balancing on one leg while pulling the foot of the other leg down the inner side.

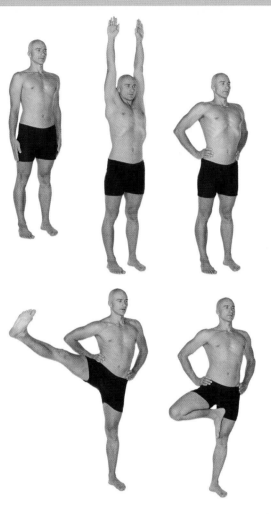

STARTING PHASE
Stand with your legs and feet parallel and your arms at your sides.

While inhaling slowly and directly, raise your arms and rotate them backward in a full circle to bring your hands on your hips with your fingers pointing forward and your thumbs backward.

CENTRAL PHASE
Holding open, extend one leg out to the side.
   In the first round, women extend the left leg and men extend the right leg.

Still holding, bring your foot to the top of the thigh of your standing leg, or as high as possible.

Still holding open, pull your foot down along your standing leg, pressing energetically all the way down to your ankle to produce a massaging effect.

Still holding, extend your leg forward with your toes pointing.

Still holding, bend your leg, raising your knee toward your abdomen.

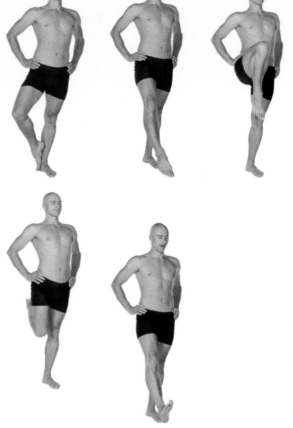

Still holding, bring your knee down and your heel up toward your buttock.

Finally, exhale forcefully with "HA," energetically kicking the foot forward and focusing the momentum on your heel. Use the strength of the exhalation to drive the movement.

REPETITION

Return to standing position with your legs parallel and your arms at your sides and repeat the sequence on the first side two more times to complete the first round. For the second round, repeat the sequence three times on the opposite side.

In the second round, women extend the right leg and men extend the left leg.

CONCLUDING PHASE

To conclude this Tsadul, inhale quickly and with strength as you raise your arms above your head.

Exhale quickly and with strength, bringing your hands to the top of your feet and your forehead to your knees. Repeat this process of inhaling quickly and dropping down as you exhale a total of three times.

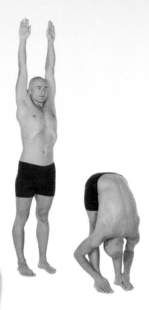

HEALTH BENEFITS
- *Alleviates ailments of the feet and legs, particularly the tendons and joints*
- *Relieves problems caused by the impaired functioning of the downward-clearing prana*

Related Warm-Ups (see Appendix 1): Tree (2)

Third Tsadul | ROTATING THE ARMS

THE THIRD TSADUL works with the upper body and ascending prana. It can also be done without the hold phase, and it works well as a warm-up for the shoulders. The succession of movements naturally facilitates a strong exhalation to fully expel the stale prana.

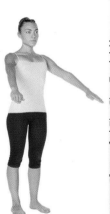

STARTING PHASE
Stand with your legs parallel and your arms at your sides.

Inhale slowly and directly, raising your arms straight and parallel along the side of your head.

CENTRAL PHASE
Holding open, energetically rotate your arms and shoulders backward three times, then forward three times.
While rotating, keep your arms tense and firmly controlled and as close as possible to your head.

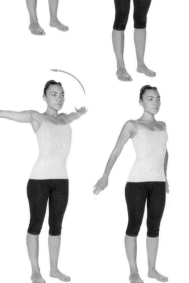

At the end of the third forward rotation, fling your arms vigorously backward and bend your torso forward a little while strongly exhaling all the stale air with "HA."

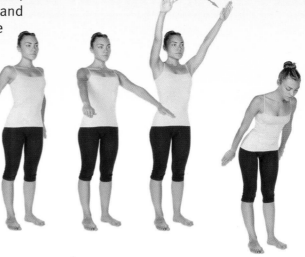

REPETITION
Repeat the entire sequence a total of three times.

CONCLUDING PHASE
To conclude this Tsadul, inhale quickly and with strength and raise your arms above your head.

Exhale quickly and with strength, bringing your hands to the top of your feet and your forehead to your knees. Repeat this process of inhaling quickly and dropping down as you exhale a total of three times.

At this point, if you like, you can stand up straight and repeat the entire exercise again. For an alternative without the hold, inhale slowly while rotating your arms backward and exhale forcefully while rotating them forward.

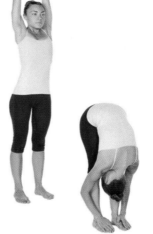

TRANSITION

Inhaling, sit on your buttocks with your knees open and the soles of your feet together while raising your arms up. Exhaling, place your hands on your knees.

HEALTH BENEFITS

- *Alleviates ailments of the muscles and ligaments of the arms and of the shoulder and elbow joints*
- *Relieves problems caused by impaired functioning of the ascending prana*
- *Keeps the shoulders flexible*
- *Opens the chest*

Fourth Tsadul | CLOSING THE ARMPITS

THE FOURTH TSADUL has a particularly strong action on the level of the channels. Perform it with vigor and intent, without restraining the force of your movements, to experience its full power.

STARTING PHASE

Sit on the floor with the soles of your feet together, knees wide apart, hands on your knees, and your back straight.

Inhaling slowly, make your hands into vajra fists and pull them firmly from your knees along your thighs and sides up to your armpits.

CENTRAL PHASE

Holding open, vigorously open your arms to the sides and immediately bend them back to hit your fists directly on top of your shoulders. Repeat three times.

Still holding open, after hitting your shoulders the third time, strike your elbows against your sides, intently closing your armpits.

Then, still holding, throw your fists straight forward, out from the shoulders.

Still holding, pull your arms back, opening your elbows outward and then striking your sides.

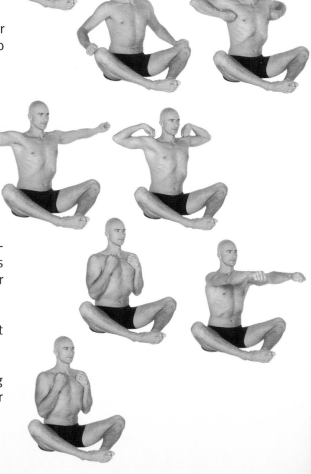

Still holding, again throw your fists straight forward.

Still holding, pull your arms back a third time, again opening your elbows outward and striking your sides.

Now exhale strongly and thoroughly with "HA" while energetically throwing your fists straight forward.

REPETITION
Bring your hands back to your knees in vajra fists and repeat the entire sequence two more times.

CONCLUDING PHASE
Inhale forcefully, raising your arms above your head while opening your legs wide apart.

Exhale forcefully, bringing your fingers to your toes and your forehead to the floor. Inhaling quickly, rise up again and bend forward to reach your toes as you exhale for a total of three times.

TRANSITION
Inhale forcefully, raising your arms above your head while keeping your legs wide apart.

Exhale energetically, bringing your hands to your knees and the soles of your feet together.

HEALTH BENEFITS
- *Relieves disorders of the shoulders and related nerves, ligaments, and joints*
- *Alleviates problems of the lungs, heart, and rib cage*

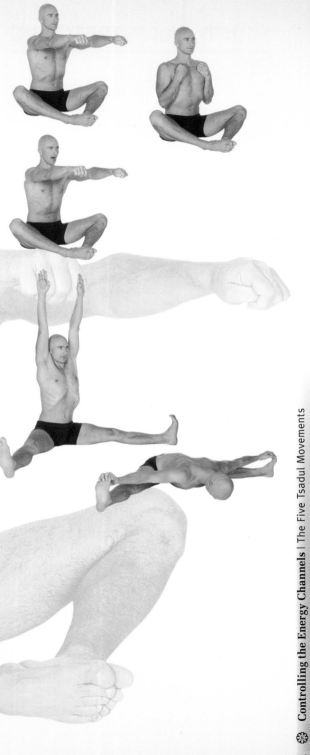

Fifth Tsadul | STRETCHING

T HE FIFTH TSADUL has a different feel from the others because the final "HA" exhalation does not come naturally with same strength and requires more active intent. It is a highly effective stretch for the spine and can also be performed without holding, simply inhaling and exhaling as you reach forward.

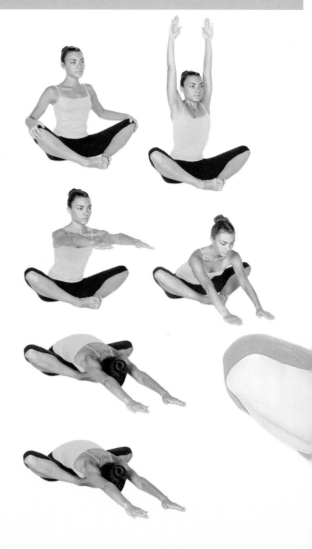

STARTING PHASE
Sit with the soles of your feet together, your knees wide apart, and your hands on your knees.

Inhaling slowly and completely, raise your arms up straight and open your chest.

CENTRAL PHASE
Holding open, first lower your extended arms to chest height, then bring them downward to touch the floor.

Still holding open, stretch your spine well, keeping it straight as you reach forward, trying to bring your forehead to the floor and your arms as far forward as possible.
  If you cannot touch the floor with your hands, simply make an effort to stretch as far as you can.

Continue to stretch forward until you reach a comfortable but challenging limit, then exhale vigorously with "HA" to expel the stale prana.

REPETITION

Return your hands to your knees and repeat the entire sequence two more times.

CONCLUDING PHASE

At the end, inhale with strength, lifting your arms up while opening your legs wide apart.

Then exhale with strength, bringing your fingers to or near your toes and your fore-head to the floor. Inhale with strength and rise up again, then bend forward to reach your toes as you exhale for a total of three times.

TRANSITION

Now you can either relax a moment by lying down with your arms out to the side and your feet slightly apart or continue with your session of practice.

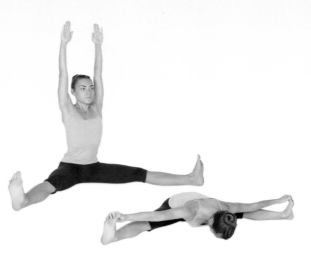

HEALTH BENEFITS

- *Alleviates ailments of the spine and the spinal cord*
- *Relieves conditions of the six hollow organs*
- *Counteracts problems caused by the impaired or disordered func-tioning of the fire-accompanying, downward-clearing, and ascending pranas*

The Five Series
of Yantras

THE TWENTY-FIVE YANTRAS, divided into five series, form the core of the practice of Yantra Yoga. The three preliminary groups—Tsigjong, Lungsang, and Tsadul—give us the tools to create a correct base, reshaping and harmonizing our body, breathing, and energy. Building on this foundation, the twenty-five Yantras further deepen and stabilize our practice, bringing to fruition our full, rich potentiality.

Unless otherwise specified in the instructions, the inhalations and exhalations in all of the Yantras are direct, long, and full. This quality can be referred to as calm breathing. The movements are always done with intent, vigor, and harmony, but without forcing or straining. Make sure you never push yourself beyond your capacity. With steady practice, the quality of your movement and breathing naturally progresses and evolves.

Each series consists of five Yantras made up of seven breathing cycles, mostly based on a rhythm of four relaxed counts synchronized with the movement and the breathing: a preliminary inhalation and exhalation; a central phase consisting of an inhalation, a specific type of retention of the breath facilitated by the unique characteristics of each Yantra, and an exhalation; and finally a concluding inhalation and exhalation. In some Yantras, a count of six is specified for the central hold, preceded or followed by a two-count phase of inhaling, exhaling, or holding empty. The holding of the air is considered the most important moment in the sequence because this is where prana can be controlled, balanced, and activated to deliver the distinct benefits indicated for each Yantra.

Each Yantra is designed to train one of five specific retentions of air or holds: open, directed, closed, contracted, and empty. The first Yantra of each of the five groups trains open hold, the second directed hold, the third closed hold, the fourth contracted hold, and the last empty hold. Open hold is when you hold without blocking or closing. The sensation is as if you want to inhale more, but are full. Nevertheless, you keep expanding, keeping open, without blocking the breathing passages in any way. When you exhale after an open hold, it should be easy and free, without any sense of constriction. Directed hold is when you direct the air downward or sideways by muscular force. It can follow an open or a closed hold. In closed hold, you contain or block the air, closing or concentrating it below the navel. In contracted hold, having closed the hold, and keeping the downward control, you draw your abdomen in toward your spine. Empty hold is when you stay empty after exhaling the air.

The key to deepening the practice is to be aware and present, to always be with the breathing, whether you are inhaling, exhaling, or holding. The body and breathing should move together as one, in total synchronicity. In the same way, individual phases of movement and breathing should be timed to start and conclude together.

In a session of personal practice, you can choose to do just one of the series of Yantras or more, depending on your capacity and the time available. You can link the individual Yantras without breaking the flow of present, relaxed breathing. The transitions have been provided to help you connect from one sequence to the next in a fluid and continuous progression, but if any of the transitions are difficult for you, you can find your way to the next starting position. You can also create your own series of five Yantras taken from any of the five different series, provided you include one Yantra for each of the five different holds and do them in the same progressive sequence (open, directed, closed, contracted, and empty). When you customize a sequence of Yantras, you can explore which of the transitions works best if you want to create a smooth passage from one to the next. A few Yantras need no specific transition since the concluding exhalation readily connects to the initial inhalation of the next Yantra.

In any yoga session, it is important to balance and compensate when practicing different asanas. In Yantra Yoga, this principle is already integrated in the sequence of each Yantra and in the sequence of the five Yantras of any given group. The structural balancing, harmonization, and compensation of the different postural challenges are embedded in the sequences themselves. It is possible, of course, that at times you will want to focus on a particular type of hold or Yantra that is challenging for you so as to deepen your understanding of it. In that case, it is best to include at least one full round of the eight Lungsang movements at the beginning and the Vajra Wave at the end of your session to counterbalance and harmonize your breathing.

Among other benefits, properly practicing the five series of Yantras restores the balance of the earth, water, fire, and air elements. The five series help the body maintain good health and overcome the various types of disturbances caused by malfunctions of the life-sustaining prana and the four other pranas. As a result of the practice, sight and the other senses become clearer and physical strength increases.

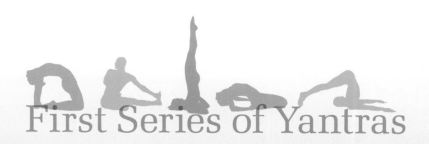

First Series of Yantras

LIKE EACH OF the five series of Yantras, the first series trains the five types of hold in succession, starting with open hold (Camel), followed by directed hold (Conch), closed hold (Flame), contracted hold (Turtle), and empty hold (Plow). All of the Yantras in the first series are based on a count of four, with the exception of the Turtle, which has a six-count contracted hold in its central phase. The first series as a whole helps train and deepen the function of open hold in particular.

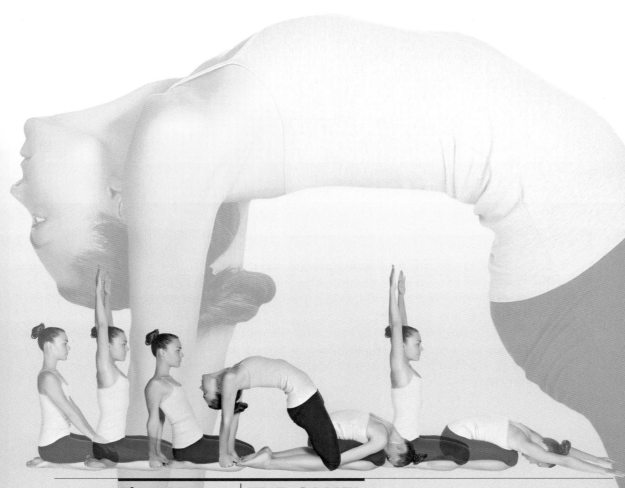

First Yantra | THE CAMEL

THE CAMEL IS the first Yantra of the first of the five series. In its central phase, it trains and facilitates a clear experience of open hold. Yantras to train open hold emphasize positions with the chest and throat open, as this promotes the full expansion of the lungs and an easy, open retention of the air. Each of the seven breathing cycles of the Camel is done in four counts. It is essential to coordinate each movement of each cycle with the count and the corresponding aspect of the breathing.

STARTING POSITION

Sit on your heels with your back straight and your hands on your knees.

If you find the position uncomfortable, you may need to place a cushion or folded blanket between your buttocks and your heels. You may also find it helpful to put a small cushion under the front of your ankles. The crucial point is to maintain the correct alignment of the spine.

INITIAL INHALATION

In four counts, extend your arms straight over your head, opening your shoulders and chest well while inhaling directly, completely, and calmly.

It is important to extend your arms well to effectively and correctly fill your lungs.

INITIAL EXHALATION

In four counts, lower your arms behind you while exhaling directly, completely, and calmly. Form fists with your hands and place them directly behind your feet, pressing your thumbs on your big toes.

If necessary, place your fists farther behind or at the sides of your feet until you become more accustomed to the position.

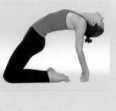

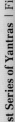

CENTRAL INHALATION

In four counts, while inhaling directly, completely, and calmly, raise your buttocks and push your chest and pelvis forward, gradually arching your spine and neck backward and assuming a shape reminiscent of a camel.

Make a point to observe whether you are really taking four counts for this movement; there can be a tendency to do it too quickly.

OPEN HOLD

For four counts, maintain the camel position while holding open. Your shoulders and chest are open and expanded, your pelvis is pushed forward, your neck is arched and relaxed back, and your throat is open.

CENTRAL EXHALATION

In four counts, exhaling directly, completely, and calmly, lower your buttocks back to your heels and bend forward with your back straight to place your forehead on the floor in front of your knees. At the same time, bring your thumbs off your toes and lay your arms on the floor along your sides.

Unlike the central inhalation, there can be a tendency to do this movement in a slower count. Here too, pay attention to performing the phase correctly in four counts, ending with your forehead on the floor.

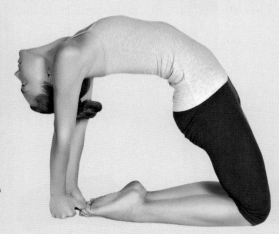

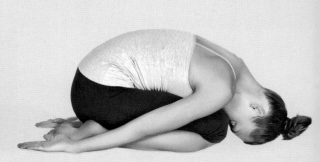

CONCLUDING INHALATION

In four counts, inhaling directly, completely, and calmly, raise your torso and extend your arms over your head, remaining seated on your heels.

Again, be sure to extend your arms well and expand your chest and shoulders so that you inhale fully and smoothly.

CONCLUDING EXHALATION

In four counts, exhaling directly, completely, and calmly and remaining seated on your heels, extend your arms forward and place your hands and forehead on the floor, with your hands outstretched and your forehead in front of your knees. Keep your arms straight to facilitate a more complete exhalation of the air.

To make this movement easier on your lower back, you can first lower your arms to chest level and then place them on the floor. This is a helpful modification for people with mild lower back issues or any issues that make it difficult to bend forward with straight arms. It will not change the dynamics of the movements or the breathing.

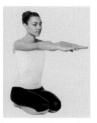

REPETITION

To enjoy the full potential of the benefits of this Yantra, repeat the entire sequence two more times, either returning to the starting position while continuing to inhale and exhale calmly, or linking the final exhalation directly to the initial inhalation of the next round.

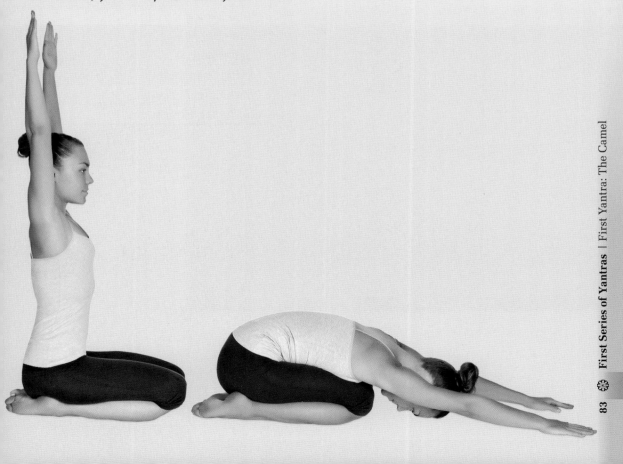

TRANSITION

To link the Camel to the starting position for the next Yantra in the first series, the Conch, inhale, coming up onto your knees with your toes curled under, and sit on your heels with your arms raised. Exhale, rolling back to sit on your buttocks while stretching your legs forward and placing your hands on your knees.

HEALTH BENEFITS

- *Invigorates the functioning of the five solid and six hollow organs*
- *Alleviates ailments of the spine and spinal cord*
- *Relieves disorders of the kidneys, lumbar region, and pelvis*
- *Improves the condition of the major and minor joints*
- *Counteracts problems related to the fire-accompanying and ascending pranas when their functioning has deteriorated or become disordered*

Related Warm-Ups (see Appendix 1): Bridge (29), Cat (31), Snake Training (33), Snake Training II (34), Neck Roll (37)

BREATHING CYCLE	COUNTS
Initial Inhalation	4
Initial Exhalation	4
Central Inhalation	4
Open Hold	**4**
Central Exhalation	4
Concluding Inhalation	4
Concluding Exhalation	4

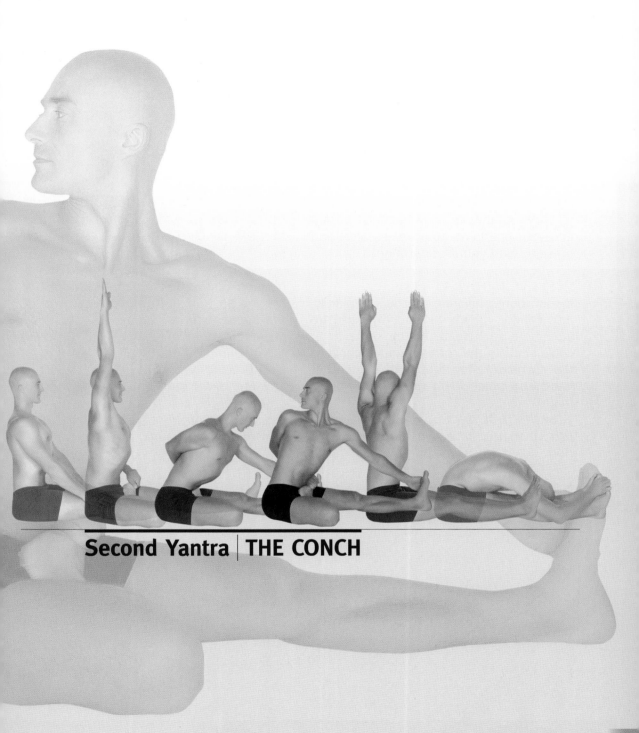

Second Yantra | THE CONCH

T HE CONCH TRAINS and facilitates a clear experience of directed hold. Directed hold is when the held air is directed either evenly downward or to one side. To achieve this characteristic function, positions for directed hold tend to include twisting movements to easily direct the air. All seven cycles of the Conch are performed to a count of four, always coordinating the movement and the breathing cycles with the rhythm of the count. As with all Yantras for directed hold, men and women start on opposite sides.

STARTING POSITION
Sit with your legs extended parallel in front and your hands on your knees, alert and present, with your back straight.

INITIAL INHALATION
In four counts, inhaling directly, completely, and calmly, slowly extend one arm up alongside your head. At the same time, while bending the corresponding leg, grab the corresponding foot with your other hand and place it on top of your other thigh.

In the first round, women raise the left arm and use the right hand to place the left foot on top of the right thigh. Men raise the right arm and use the left hand to place the right foot on top of the left thigh.

It is important to coordinate the extending of the arm and the bending of the leg so that both movements end at the same time as the completion of the inhalation. If it is difficult to bring your foot to the top of the thigh, you 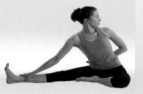 can place it on the floor with your heel next to your perineum.

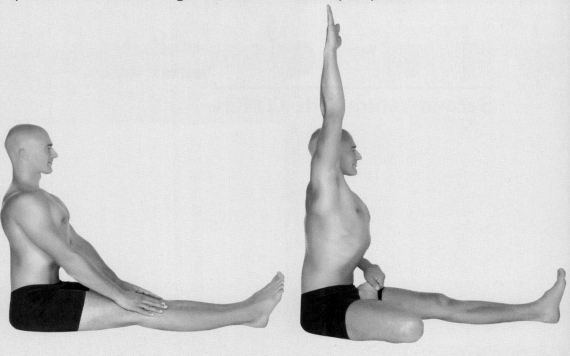

INITIAL EXHALATION

Exhaling directly, completely, and calmly in four counts, lower your raised arm and wrap it around your back to grasp the inside of the foot on the thigh from behind, then bend forward to grasp the outside of the extended foot with your other hand.

In the first round, women reach back with the left arm and bend to grab the left foot on top of the right thigh. Men reach back with the right arm and bend to grab the right foot on top of the left thigh.

If you cannot reach the foot from behind, simply reach around the back as far as possible. If you cannot bend enough to reach the outside of the foot of your extended leg, or if you have your foot on the floor next to your perineum, it is better to simply grasp the ankle of your extended leg or place your palm on the inside of your shin. In this way you can keep your spine in the correct position for the inhalation and subsequent directed hold.

CENTRAL INHALATION

In four counts, inhaling directly, completely, and calmly from below, straighten your torso upward and twist to the open side, keeping your extended arm and extended leg straight as you pull your foot toward you with your back straight and aligned.

In the first round, women turn to the left side and men turn to the right.

DIRECTED HOLD

Applying directed hold for four counts, pull your shoulder on the open side a bit farther back and look straight over it while maintaining the correct alignment of your spine and neck. Stay in this position, twisted like a conch, for the remainder of the four counts.

In the first round, women look over the left shoulder and men look over the right shoulder.

The action of the movement and position automatically directs the held air down, mainly to the open side, thus applying and training directed hold.

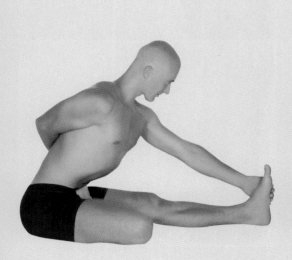
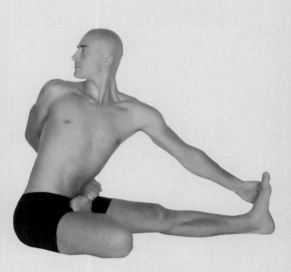

CENTRAL EXHALATION

In four counts, exhale directly, completely, and calmly, slowly extending your bent leg forward and resting your hands on your knees.

CONCLUDING INHALATION

Inhaling in four counts, extend your arms up and over your head as you gradually turn to the opposite side for a countertwist, keeping your arms alongside your head and your sides stretched and controlled.

In the first round, women twist to the right side and men twist to the left.

This movement compensates and harmoniously balances the opposite twist applied during the directed hold. Be sure to stretch well to keep the chest and glottis open and allow a smooth flow of the breathing.

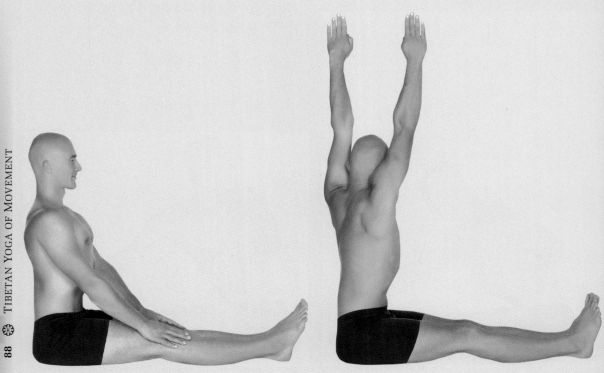

CONCLUDING EXHALATION

In four counts, exhale evenly as you bend forward, starting from the root of your spine, and lower your forehead to your knees, bringing your fingers to your toes.

REPETITION

Repeat the entire sequence on the opposite side, either returning to the starting position while continuing to inhale and exhale calmly, or linking the final exhalation directly to the initial inhalation of the second round. Then continue as before, but reversing the position of the arms and legs.

In the second round, women raise the right arm and use the left hand to place the right foot on top of the left thigh. Men raise the left arm and use the right hand to place the left foot on the top of the right thigh.

TRANSITION

To link the Conch to the next Yantra in the first series, the Flame, inhale, rising back up from the concluding exhalation while stretching your arms parallel up from your shoulders and over your head. Then exhale calmly and fully and place your hands on your knees.

HEALTH BENEFITS

- *Alleviates ailments of the kidneys*
- *Tones the ligaments of the lumbar region*
- *Relieves gout and arthritis*
- *Improves conditions related to the six hollow organs*
- *Strengthens the liver*
- *Alleviates digestive disorders arising from cold phlegm energy*
- *Counteracts problems resulting from irregular functioning of the downward-clearing prana*

Related Warm-Ups (see Appendix 1): Swinging (1), Knees to the Side (10), Knee to the Side Forward Bend (12), Crossed Knee Stretch (17), Gentle Spine Twist (21), Supine Twist (27), Neck Roll (37)

BREATHING CYCLE	COUNTS
Initial Inhalation	4
Initial Exhalation	4
Central Inhalation	4
Directed Hold	**4**
Central Exhalation	4
Concluding Inhalation	4
Concluding Exhalation	4

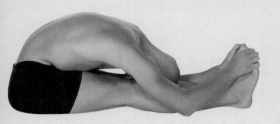

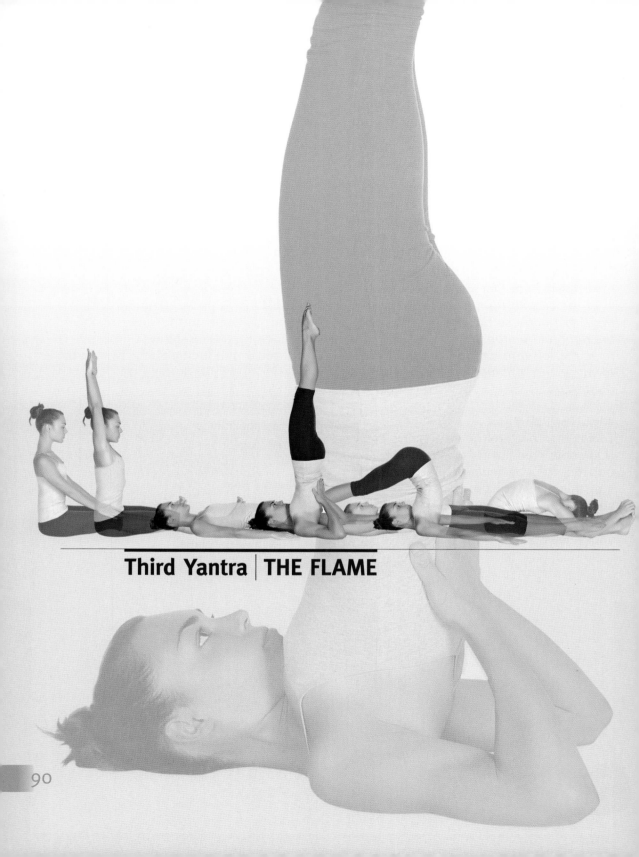

Third Yantra | THE FLAME

THE FLAME TRAINS and facilitates a clear experience of closed hold. The hold is felt as an increase in pressure below the navel as the air is first pushed downward and then locked. Positions to train closed hold tend to have the chin closed against the chest to help focus the hold below the navel and prevent the hold from creating pressure at the head and heart, both of which are contraindicated.

As in the previous Yantra, the seven breathing cycles of the Flame are all performed to a count of four, coordinated with the movement and breathing. If you have problems with your cervical vertebrae, it is of paramount importance to be especially careful with this Yantra or to substitute it with a closed hold Yantra from one of the other series.

STARTING POSITION

Sit with your legs extended and parallel, your hands resting on your knees, and your back erect and in alignment.

INITIAL INHALATION

In four counts, extend your arms upward alongside your head, inhaling fully and directly while opening and expanding your shoulders and your chest.

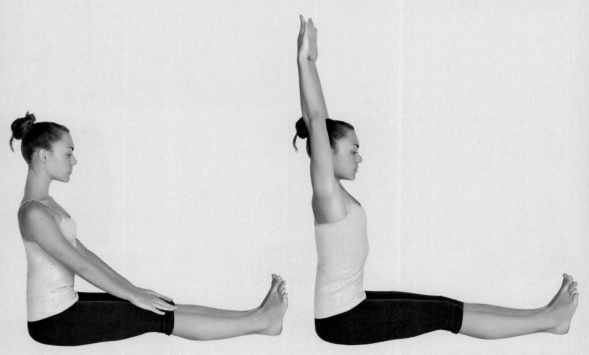

INITIAL EXHALATION

In four counts, exhale fully and directly, rolling down on your back and coming into a supine position with your arms along your sides.

CENTRAL INHALATION

In four counts, inhaling fully and directly from the bottom up, raise your feet, legs, and pelvis. Keep them controlled during the movement to come into an inverted position, aligned with your spine straight. Support your back with your hands to help straighten the spine and extend your legs up with your toes pointed upward.

If it is difficult to lift your legs straight into the air, you can bend them slightly to help yourself come up. You can also support your back with your arms at a more open angle while keeping your 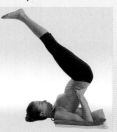 *legs straight and your feet in a line above your head. To help protect your neck, you can place padding such as a folded blanket under your shoulders and mid-cervical region, keeping your head off the padding.*

The dynamics of the movement determine the correct function of the breathing. If you have to bend your legs toward your chest to rise up into the position, it is advisable to take a soft, not full, inhalation and try to concentrate it mostly in the abdomen. This will make the application of the hold easier and more correct.

CLOSED HOLD

For four counts, hold closed as you continue to extend upward, keeping your feet, legs, and knees in straight alignment like a rising flame.

The weight of your body is mainly supported on the back of your head and shoulders with the help of your upper arms. Your chin is closed against your sternum to avoid pressure on your head. Even though you are upside down, the pressure of the held air should be felt below the navel. If you focus your inhalation mainly in the abdomen, and as long as the movement is performed in a controlled and correct manner, this condition will be created naturally.

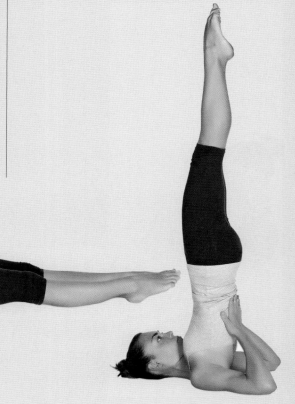

CENTRAL EXHALATION

In four counts, exhale fully and calmly while gradually lowering your legs to the floor behind your head, bringing your toes to the floor and stretching your arms out behind you.

Keep your legs straight when you lower them over your head. To make it easier, you can put your arms on the floor first. If you cannot reach the floor with your toes, simply go as far as you are able without bending your legs.

CONCLUDING INHALATION

In four counts, directly and calmly inhale while gradually swinging your arms above your head and rolling down on your spine to bring your legs back in front.

If possible, keep your arms and legs straight and have them cross past each other midway as you come into the supine position. To make it easier on your back and give yourself more support, you can keep your arms along your sides as you bring your legs to the floor and then bring them over your head. At this point, you can also bend your legs a little to make the movement even easier.

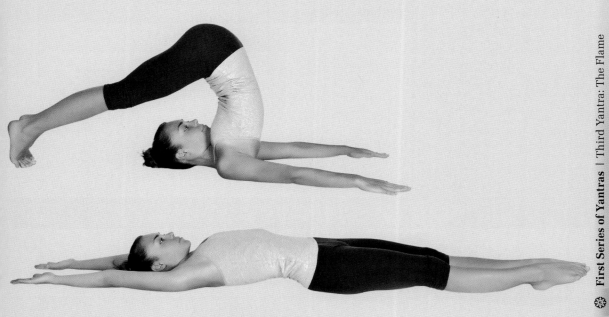

CONCLUDING EXHALATION

In four counts, while exhaling calmly, come up and ease into a forward bend, originating the movement from the base of your spine and bringing your forehead to your knees and fingers to your toes.

To make the movement easier on your lower back, you can first bring your hands to hip level and then push yourself up and bend forward. If, for any reason, the forward bending is too challenging, you can simply straighten your back and place your hands on your knees.

REPETITION

To enjoy the full potential of the benefits of this Yantra, repeat the entire sequence two more times, either returning to the starting position while continuing to inhale and exhale calmly, or linking the final exhalation directly to the initial inhalation of the next round.

TRANSITION

To link the Flame to the next Yantra in the first series, the Turtle, inhale, rising back up from the concluding exhalation and stretching your arms over your head. Then exhale and place your hands on your knees.

HEALTH BENEFITS

- *Relieves ailments of the spine and spinal cord*
- *Eases lumbar pain*
- *Improves conditions such as sciatic pain, numbness, and tingling*
- *Alleviates all types of ailments related to imbalances of wind energy*
- *Counteracts problems caused by impaired functioning of the ascending and fire-accompanying pranas*

Related Warm-Ups (see Appendix 1): Perpendicular Leg Stretch (24), Spine Roll (30)

BREATHING CYCLE	COUNTS
Initial Inhalation	4
Initial Exhalation	4
Central Inhalation	4
Closed Hold	**4**
Central Exhalation	4
Concluding Inhalation	4
Concluding Exhalation	4

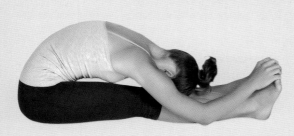

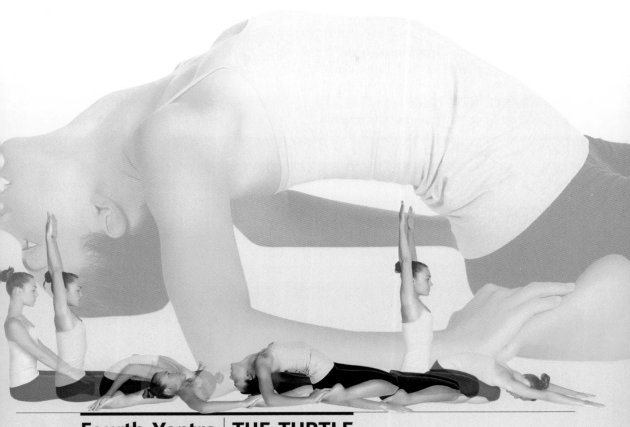

Fourth Yantra | **THE TURTLE**

THE TURTLE TRAINS contracted hold, facilitating a clear experience of it in its central phase. In contracted hold, after concentrating and controlling the air downward, the abdominal muscles are contracted and pulled in toward the spine. It is the first Yantra to include a count of two and six in addition to counts of four.

The Turtle is a difficult position for many people. Using padding as described below can help, but if you have knee problems, it is best to substitute it with one of the fourth Yantras from another series, such as the Dog or the Tiger.

STARTING POSITION
Sit with your legs forward and parallel, your back correctly aligned, and your hands resting on your knees.

INITIAL INHALATION
In four counts, inhale directly, completely, and calmly and raise your arms over your head, keeping them straight and extending them well.

It is important to extend your arms well to allow your lungs to fill correctly and help your chest expand to its full capacity.

INITIAL EXHALATION
In four counts, exhale directly, completely, and calmly while bringing your heels toward your perineum, rolling onto your knees, and bending forward to bring your forehead to the floor in front of your knees and your palms to the soles of your feet.

As you come to your knees, separate your lower legs a little to sit between them. You can make the forward rolling movement easier by crossing your feet and coming up onto your knees in that way. If the movement is still an obstacle, you can help yourself into a simple kneeling position with your back straight

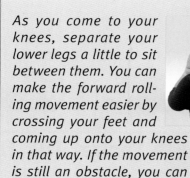

and your hands on your knees and continue the movement as described for the second and third rounds, as described in the repetition instructions below.

CENTRAL INHALATION
In four counts, inhale completely and smoothly as you raise your torso up, lean back, and come to lie flat on the floor, turning your palms around so that your thumbs are joined with your big toes.

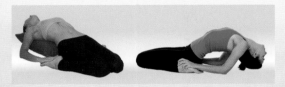

To make the position easier and more comfortable, you can place padding, such as a folded blanket, under your buttocks and your back. You can also lean back and support yourself on your elbows rather than lying flat on your back.

CONTRACTED HOLD
Quickly and forcefully sound an aspirated "HA," emptying your chest and blocking the air below the navel. Push your chest out and arch your neck back as you bring the top of your head to the floor. Then stay in a contracted hold for six counts, drawing in your sides and abdomen and forming a shape like a turtle.

Blocking the air downward and contracting the sides and abdomen toward the spine will help you train and experience the precise condition of contracted hold.

CENTRAL EXHALATION
In two counts, exhale the remaining air as you lower your back and the back of your head to the floor, relaxing all tension.

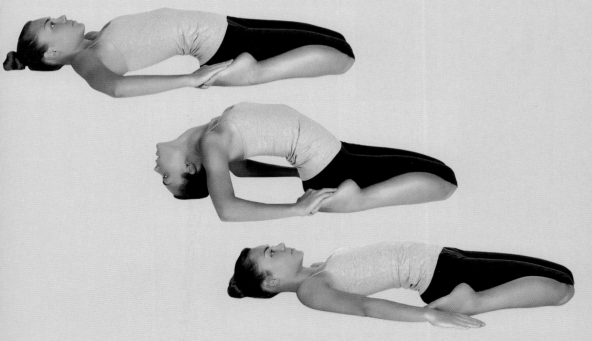

CONCLUDING INHALATION

In four counts, inhale fully and calmly and come up to sit on your heels with your legs together and your arms extended above your head.

You may need to help yourself up by placing your hands behind the small of your back and giving yourself a push. In this way, you can avoid any strain in the movement and the breathing.

CONCLUDING EXHALATION

In four counts, exhaling directly, completely, and calmly and remaining seated on your heels, extend your arms forward and place your hands and forehead on the floor, with your arms outstretched and forehead in front of your knees.

As with the Camel, to make the movement easier on your lower back, you can first lower your arms to chest level and then place them on the floor.

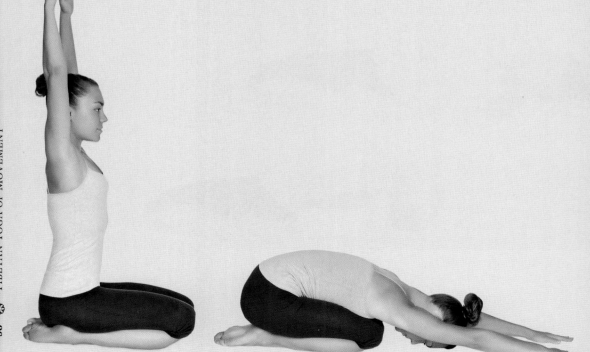

REPETITION

To enjoy the full potential of the benefits of this Yantra, repeat the entire sequence two more times. In this case, the second and third rounds start from the kneeling position, seated on your heels, with your back straight and your hands on your knees.

To begin the second and third rounds, inhale directly, completely, and calmly in four counts, rising up onto your knees and separating your lower legs a little. Then exhale in four counts, sitting between your legs and bringing your forehead to the floor in front of your knees and your palms on the soles of your feet. Now continue the sequence from the central inhalation, starting by raising your torso up to lean back and lie flat on the floor.

TRANSITION

To link the Turtle in a sequence to the starting position for the next Yantra in the first series, the Plow, inhale, coming up onto your knees with your toes curled under and sitting on your heels with your arms raised. Exhale, rolling back to sit on your buttocks while stretching your legs forward and placing your hands on your knees.

HEALTH BENEFITS

- *Alleviates chest and liver pain*
- *Tonifies the nerves of the solid and hollow organs if they are damaged and weakened*
- *Relieves disturbances of the phlegm and blood energy presenting symptoms such as difficult digestion, hyperacidity, and ulcers*

Related Warm-Ups (see Appendix 1): Hip and Knee Relaxer (11), Knee Bend (16), Transition Training (22), Hip Releaser (26)

BREATHING CYCLE	COUNTS
Initial Inhalation	4
Initial Exhalation	4
Central Inhalation	4
Contracted Hold	**6**
Central Exhalation	2
Concluding Inhalation	4
Concluding Exhalation	4

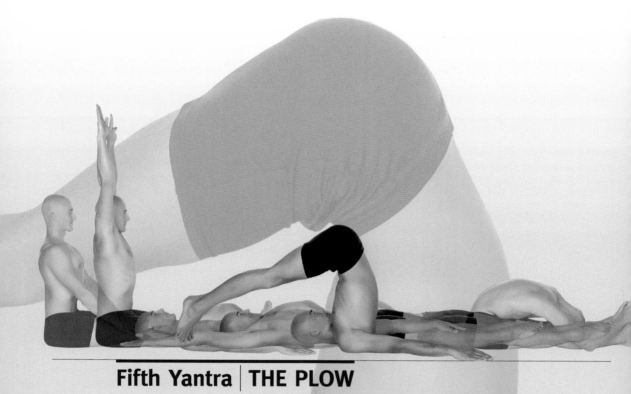

Fifth Yantra | THE PLOW

THE PLOW IS for training and experiencing empty hold. In the central phase, after thoroughly exhaling the air, you simply wait and remain empty before inhaling again. That is the condition of empty hold. In this Yantra, the central hold is a four-count pause between exhaling and inhaling.

STARTING POSITION
Sit with your legs extended and parallel. Your hands rest on your knees and your back is erect and in alignment.

INITIAL INHALATION
In four counts, extend your arms upward alongside your head, inhaling fully and directly while opening and expanding your chest and your shoulders.

INITIAL EXHALATION
In four counts, exhale fully and directly while lying on your back with your arms along your sides.

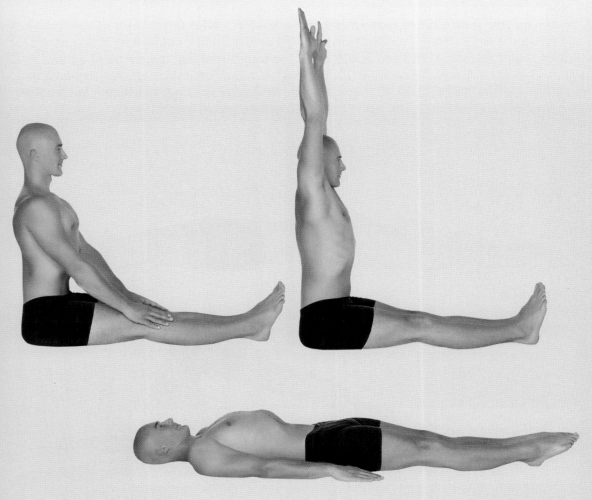

CENTRAL INHALATION

In four counts, inhaling fully and directly, swing your arms above your head, parallel and straight, and extend your toes downward, strongly tensing your whole body by stretching your arms and legs in opposite directions.

CENTRAL EXHALATION

In four counts, exhale fully and calmly as you slowly bring your arms forward and your legs back in a synchronized movement without bending your limbs. End the four counts with your feet extended beyond your head with your toes to the floor and your arms stretched out behind your back.

If you find it difficult to reach the floor with your toes pointed, you can curl your toes under instead. If this too is difficult,

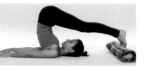

you can use a support like a rolled blanket, a prop, or a chair to help keep your legs straight while allowing you to correctly apply the empty hold, optionally also placing a small mat or thick blanket at your mid-cervical region with your head

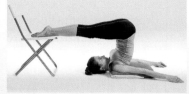

off the mat and on the floor. If you cannot keep your legs straight, you can bend your legs a little.

EMPTY HOLD

For four counts, hold empty in this position, which resembles the shape of a plow.

Do not force yourself into this position. Be careful not to push yourself farther than your capacity allows.

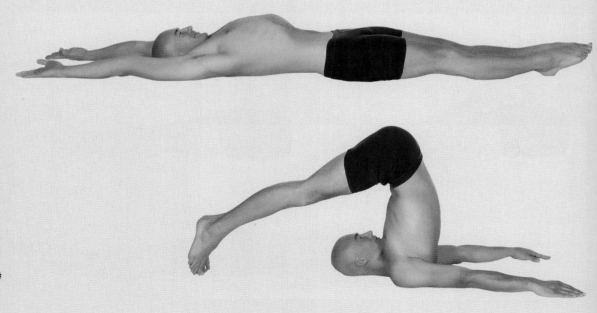

CONCLUDING INHALATION

In four counts, inhale directly and calmly while swinging your arms above your head and your legs back in front in a synchronized movement similar to the concluding inhalation of the Flame.

To make it easier on your back, you can keep your arms on the floor along your sides to help swing your legs forward without effort and then bring your arms over your head. You can also bend your legs a little to make the movement even easier.

CONCLUDING EXHALATION

In four counts, exhaling directly, completely, and calmly, come up and ease into a forward bend with your forehead to your knees and your fingers to your toes.

If needed, you can make the movement easier on your lower back by first bringing your hands to hip level and then helping yourself rise to come into the forward bend.

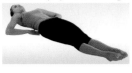

REPETITION

To enjoy the full potential of the benefits of this Yantra, repeat the entire sequence two more times, either returning to the starting position while continuing to inhale and exhale calmly, or linking the final exhalation directly to the initial inhalation of the next round.

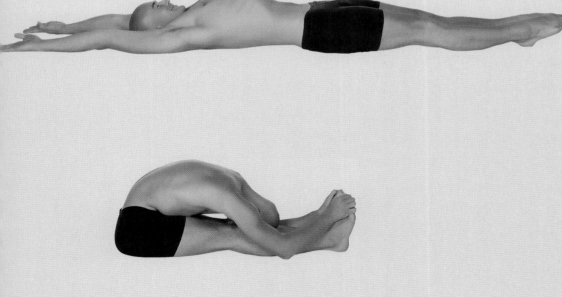

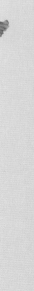

TRANSITION

If you are doing the first and second series in a single session, you can link the Plow to the first Yantra of the second series, the Snake. To connect the two series in a continuous sequence, inhale slowly and directly and raise your arms over your head. While exhaling slowly and directly, bring your heels toward your perineum, lower your arms, and roll forward onto your knees to sit on your heels with the tops of your feet flat on the floor and your hands resting on your knees.

If you find it difficult to roll forward onto your knees, you can cross your legs at the ankles as you roll forward, as in the transition to the fourth Tsigjong and the beginning of the fourth Lungsang.

HEALTH BENEFITS

- *Alleviates ailments of the spine and spinal cord*
- *Relieves conditions of the five solid and six hollow organs*
- *Counteracts problems related to the ligaments of the head and limbs*
- *Strengthens and restores the balance of the five pranas when their functions are impaired or weakened*

Related Warm-Ups (see Appendix 1): Perpendicular Leg Stretch (24), Hip Opener (28), Spine Roll (30)

Breathing Cycle	Counts
Initial Inhalation	4
Initial Exhalation	4
Central Inhalation	4
Central Exhalation	4
Empty Hold	4
Concluding Inhalation	4
Concluding Exhalation	4

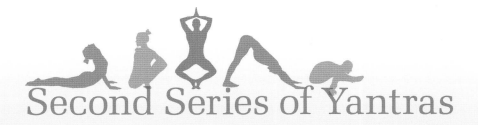

Second Series of Yantras

IN THE SECOND series, the Snake is for open hold, the Curved Knife for directed hold, the Dagger for closed hold, the Dog for contracted hold, and the Spider for empty hold. A unique aspect of the first four Yantras of this series is that in the exhalation after the central hold, we exhale for only two counts and then remain in empty hold for two counts. In the fourth and fifth Yantras, the central hold is for six counts. The second series as a whole helps train and deepen the function of directed hold in particular.

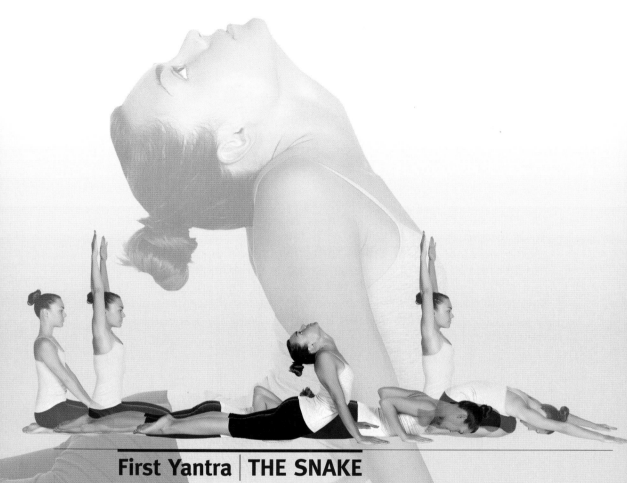

First Yantra | THE SNAKE

THE SNAKE IS for the experience, training, and application of open hold. Open hold is simply allowing the air to keep expanding in the lungs without blocking the glottis or any part of the breathing passages. It is a retention of the air with an experience of freedom from tension; free from the common habit of blocking, tensing, or fragmenting the flow of our breath. We hold, but with an open feeling. It is important to notice how this openness is experienced. Surprisingly, it comes about when we are thoroughly tensing our whole body. We actually use this body tension, this strength, to help keep the hold open, to keep the space inside free from blocking. All seven breathing cycles of the Snake are done in four counts.

STARTING POSITION

Sit on your heels with your spine erect and your hands on your knees. Your mind is present and focused, and your breathing is calm and relaxed.

If needed, you can use some cushioning between your buttocks and your heels or under your ankles to facilitate the position.

INITIAL INHALATION

In four counts, extend your arms straight over your head, opening your shoulders and chest well while inhaling directly, completely, and calmly.

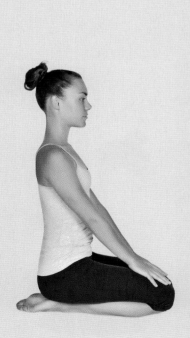
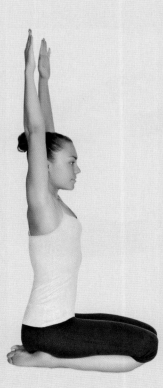

INITIAL EXHALATION

First exhale for two counts while fully stretching your arms forward and placing your palms and forehead on the floor.

Stretching forward as far as you can reach will bring your hands into the right position for the next step.

Then complete the next two counts of the exhalation as you lie on your abdomen, keeping your palms on the floor alongside your chest, with your pelvis, chin, and throat firmly on the floor. Your legs are energetically extended with your feet and big toes close together.

CENTRAL INHALATION

In four counts, while inhaling directly, lift and arch your head back as you raise and open your chest and straighten your elbows without lifting the lower part of your body from the floor. Your chest is expanded and your shoulders are open. Keep your lower pubis on the floor.

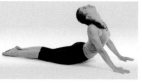

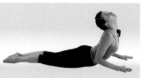

You may have to place your hands a little farther forward to be able to straighten your arms. If it is still difficult, you can also bend your arms a little so you can keep your pelvis on the floor. In this Yantra, the body tension stabilizes and protects the condition of the spine while allowing a better expansion of the held air. The improved expansion of the open hold, in turn, further helps to protect and stabilize the spine.

OPEN HOLD

For four counts, remain in the position of the Snake in the full expansion of open hold while tensing all the muscles and nerves of your body, thoroughly stretching from head to toes.

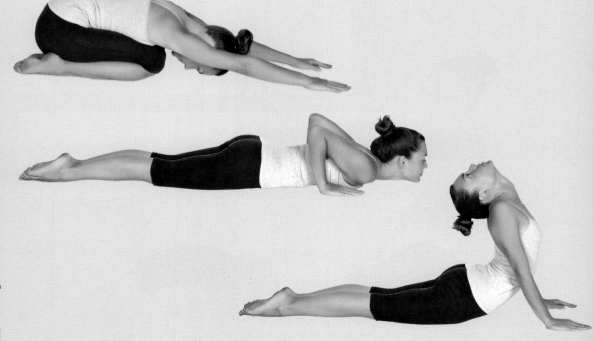

The complete tension of this phase helps stabilize and protect the back. Be sure that your shoulders are open, the back of your head is arched, and you have not closed your throat in any way.

CENTRAL EXHALATION
Exhale quickly in two counts, lowering your torso and forehead to the floor, and then remain empty for two counts.

CONCLUDING INHALATION
In four counts, inhaling directly, completely, and calmly, come up to sit on your heels and extend your arms parallel over your head.

CONCLUDING EXHALATION
In four counts, exhaling directly, completely, and calmly, lower your forehead and palms to the floor in front of you with your arms outstretched.

As with the Camel, you can bring your arms straight down to the floor or first lower them to chest level and then bend forward to extend them on the floor.

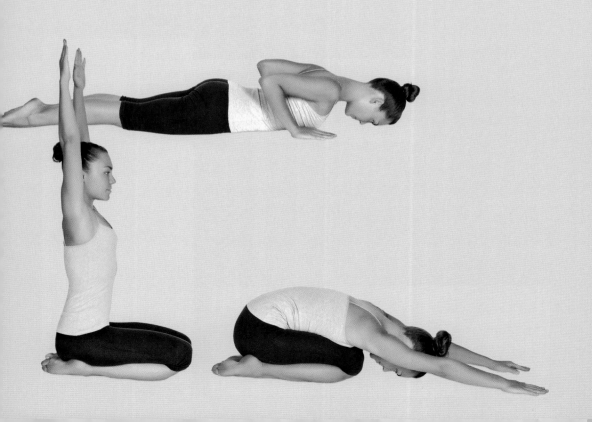

REPETITION

To enjoy the full potential of the benefits of this Yantra, repeat the entire sequence two more times, either returning to the starting position while continuing to inhale and exhale calmly, or linking the final exhalation directly to the initial inhalation of the next round.

TRANSITION

To link the Snake to the starting position of the next Yantra in the second series, the Curved Knife, inhale, coming up to sit on your heels with your toes curled under and your arms raised. Exhale, rolling back to sit on your buttocks while stretching your legs forward and placing your hands on your knees.

HEALTH BENEFITS

- *Alleviates ailments of the spine and spinal cord*
- *Improves the condition of the major and minor joints*
- *Relieves disorders related to the ligaments of the head and limbs*
- *Alleviates ailments of the five solid and six hollow organs*
- *Counteracts problems caused by the impaired functioning of the five pranas*

Related Warm-Ups (see Appendix 1): Snake Training (33), Snake Training II (34), Neck Roll (37)

BREATHING CYCLE		COUNTS
Initial Inhalation		4
Initial Exhalation		4
Central Inhalation		4
Open Hold		**4**
Central Exhalation	Exhalation	2
	Empty Hold	2
Concluding Inhalation		4
Concluding Exhalation		4

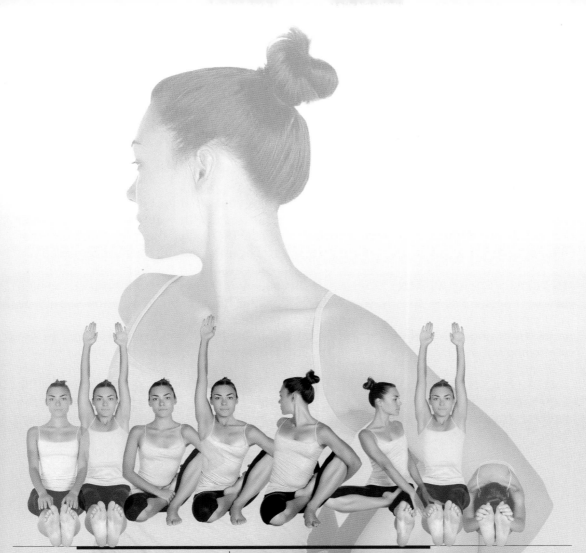

Second Yantra | THE CURVED KNIFE

THE CURVED KNIFE is for applying, experiencing, and training directed hold. This position, like the Conch, is characterized by a twist that causes most of the retained air to be pushed or directed to one side. It trains our bodies to open to more complete and relaxed breathing. All seven breathing cycles are done in four counts. Men and women start on opposite sides.

STARTING POSITION
Sit with your legs forward and your hands on your knees with your spine upright and aligned.

INITIAL INHALATION
In four counts, inhaling directly, completely, and calmly, extend your arms up, opening your chest and your shoulders well and stretching your spine.

INITIAL EXHALATION
Exhaling in four counts, bring one foot to your groin on top of your thigh with the corresponding hand and place your other foot in front of it, close to your body, with your knee raised to your chest. Then place the armpit of your other arm over the front of the raised knee as you reach around to the back with that hand, making a vajra fist. Both buttocks remain on the floor, and the position should be stable.

In the first round, women bring the right foot to the groin using the right hand, raise the left knee, and place the left armpit over the raised knee while reaching around the back with the left arm. Men bring the left foot to the groin using the left hand, raise the right knee, and place the right armpit over the raised knee while reaching around the back with the right arm.

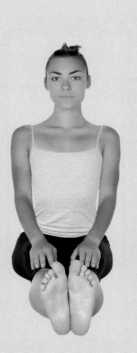
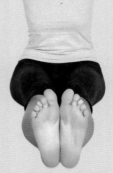
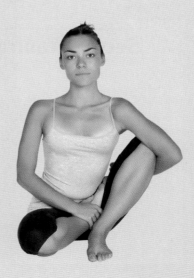

You may need to place your foot in front of your perineum on the floor rather than bringing it to your groin in order to keep your back straight and your buttocks on the floor.

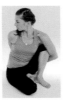

CENTRAL INHALATION

In four counts, inhaling directly and completely, slowly raise the hand that is resting on your foot, synchronizing the movement so that the inhalation ends when your arm is fully stretched up.

In the first round, women raise the right arm and men raise the left arm.

DIRECTED HOLD

Then, in four counts, lower your arm and wrap it around your back to grab your fist above the wrist while applying directed hold as you turn your torso and head to 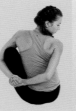 the open side.
Maintain this position, which resembles a curved knife, for the remainder of the count.

In the first round, women turn to the right and men turn to the left.

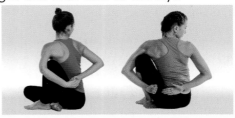

You can also grab just your fingers, or reach around as far as you can. The held air is automatically directed by the movement of twisting to the open side (the side with the knee on the floor).

CENTRAL EXHALATION

In two counts, lower your raised knee to the floor as you extend your leg forward while twisting to the opposite side. Place your hands on the floor by that side and remain empty for two more counts.

In the first round, women extend the left leg forward and turn to the left; men extend the right leg forward and turn to the right.

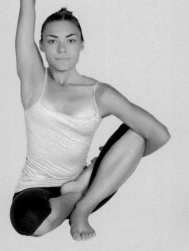

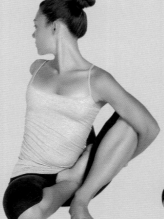

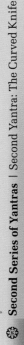

CONCLUDING INHALATION

Inhaling fully and directly in four counts, turn to the front as you extend your arms over your head.

CONCLUDING EXHALATION

In four counts, exhale as you bend forward, starting the movement from the root of your spine, and bring your forehead to your knees and your fingers to your toes.

REPETITION

Repeat the entire sequence on the opposite side, either returning to the starting position while continuing to inhale and exhale calmly, or linking the final exhalation directly to the initial inhalation of the second round. Then continue as before, but reversing the position of your arms and legs.

In the second round, women bring the left foot to the groin using the left hand, raise the right knee, and place the right armpit over the raised knee while reaching around the back with the right arm. Men bring the right foot to the groin using the right hand, raise the left knee, and place the left armpit over the raised knee while reaching around the back with the left arm.

TRANSITION

To link the Curved Knife to the next Yantra in the second series, the Dagger, inhale, rising back up from the concluding exhalation and stretching your arms over your head. Then exhale and place your hands on your knees.

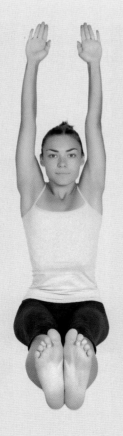
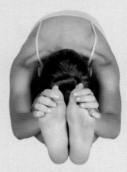

HEALTH BENEFITS

- *Alleviates kidney ailments*
- *Relieves pain in the joints of the lumbosacral region*
- *Counteracts problems related to imbalances of phlegm energy*
- *Improves digestive problems such as the accumulation of mucus in the stomach, lack of appetite, and difficult digestion*
- *Relieves asthma and other respiratory problems*
- *Counteracts conditions caused by disorders of the fire-accompanying and downward-clearing pranas*

Related Warm-Ups (see Appendix 1): Swinging (1), Knees to the Chest (9), Knees to the Side (10), Knee to the Side Forward Bend (12), Knee over Knee (18), Supine Twist (27), Hip Opener (28), Shoulder and Chest Opener (39)

BREATHING CYCLE		COUNTS
Initial Inhalation		4
Initial Exhalation		4
Central Inhalation		4
Directed Hold		**4**
Central Exhalation	Exhalation	2
	Empty Hold	2
Concluding Inhalation		4
Concluding Exhalation		4

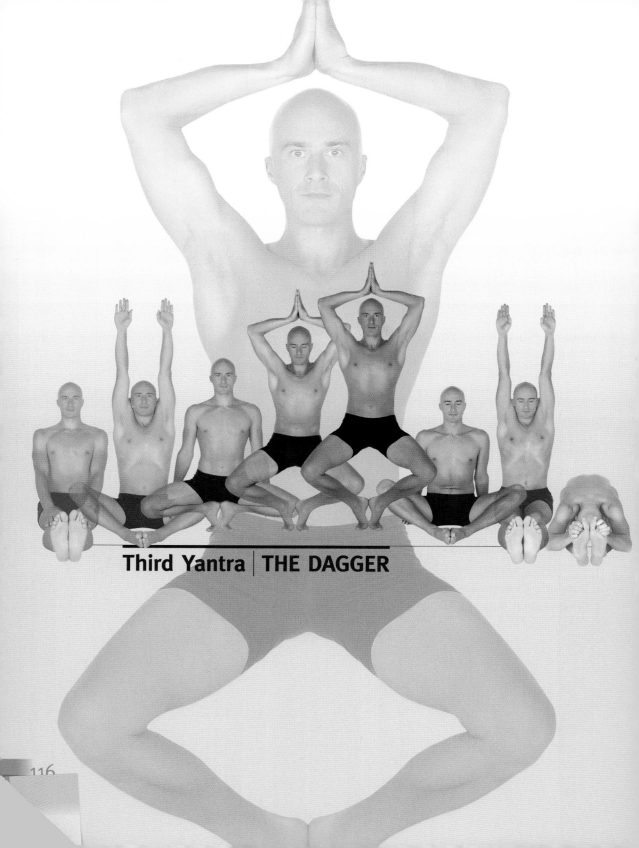

Third Yantra | **THE DAGGER**

116

THE DAGGER IS for developing and experiencing closed hold. It effectively trains the body how to enter this type of hold smoothly and correctly. The dynamics of the position facilitate the downward blocking of the air. In this case, there is a progression from open hold through directed hold into a closed hold, where the air is concentrated downward and the pressure felt below the navel. All seven breathing cycles are done in four counts. The breathing is direct, full, and relaxed.

STARTING POSITION
Sit with your legs stretched forward and your hands on your knees. Your spine is straight and erect, and you are present and alert yet relaxed.

INITIAL INHALATION
In four counts, inhaling directly, completely, and calmly, stretch your arms over your head as you open the shoulders, fully expand your chest, and straighten your spine.

At the same time, bring your heels to your perineum with the soles of your feet joined and your knees wide apart.

INITIAL EXHALATION
Exhaling directly and fully in four counts, lower your arms by your sides while rolling up onto your toes, trying to bring your heels together.

You may need to help yourself up with your hands, pushing from behind.

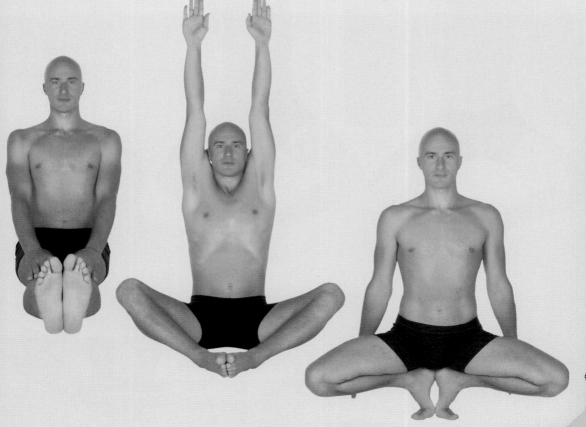

CENTRAL INHALATION

Inhaling in four counts directly and completely, starting from below, raise your arms and open your shoulders and elbows to bring your palms tightly pressed together just above your head in line with the crown of your head. At the same time, rise up on your toes, keeping your heels together and your knees and elbows wide apart.

Avoid rising up too far, as otherwise the Yantra loses its characteristic function to correctly shape the closed hold.

CLOSED HOLD

Holding for four counts, rise up a little more. Push your pelvis slightly forward and stretch and align your spine well while applying, in succession, open hold, followed by directed hold, and finally locking into closed hold as you stay in this position, which resembles a dagger.

CENTRAL EXHALATION

In two counts, exhale quickly while gently sitting back down on the floor, letting your hands come to the floor by your sides and remaining empty and relaxed for two more counts, with your back straight.

CONCLUDING INHALATION

In four counts, inhale directly and calmly while raising your arms over your head, opening your shoulders and chest, and stretching your legs forward.

CONCLUDING EXHALATION

In four counts, exhale calmly while bringing your forehead to your knees and your fingers to your toes.

Be aware of lengthening and aligning your spine correctly.

REPETITION

To enjoy the full potential of the benefits of this Yantra, repeat the entire sequence two more times, either returning to the starting position while continuing to inhale and exhale calmly, or linking the final exhalation directly to the initial inhalation of the next round.

TRANSITION

To link the Dagger to the next Yantra in the second series, the Dog, inhale and raise your arms over your head. Exhaling, bring your heels toward your perineum while lowering your arms and rolling forward onto your knees to sit on your heels with the tops of your feet flat on the floor and your hands resting on your knees.

You can also cross your legs to roll forward into the kneeling position.

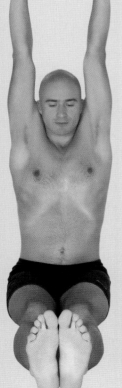

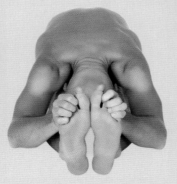

HEALTH BENEFITS
- *Alleviates illnesses of the upper and lower torso*
- *Counteracts problems of the tendons and ligaments of the head, arms, and legs*
- *Rebalances the earth, water, fire, and air elements of the body*
- *Harmonizes the various energies linked with the voice and mind*
- *Increases physical strength*

Related Warm-Ups (see Appendix 1): Squat (3), Transition Training (22), Perpendicular Leg Stretch (24), Hip Opener (28)

BREATHING CYCLE		COUNTS	
Initial Inhalation		4	
Initial Exhalation		4	
Central Inhalation		4	
Closed Hold		**4**	
Central Exhalation	Exhalation	2	
	Empty Hold	2	
Concluding Inhalation		4	
Concluding Exhalation		4	

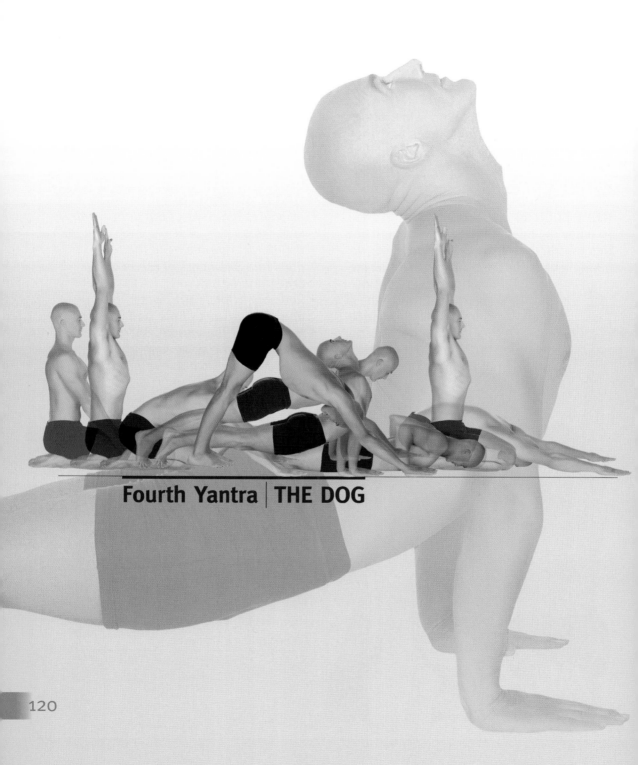

Fourth Yantra | **THE DOG**

THE DOG IS for training and applying contracted hold. As in the Turtle, the Yantra for contracted hold in the first series, some air is blocked below the navel after partially exhaling from the mouth with a short "HA" sound. The air from the top is expelled while the abdominal muscles are pulled back, thus trapping and pulling back the held air, which is felt below the navel.

In the Dog, we inhale for two counts in the central phase, then block the air with "HA" and apply the contracted hold for six counts. Then, as for all Yantras in the second series, we exhale for two counts and remain empty for two counts. For many people, the Dog is one of the easier positions for contracted hold and can be substituted for any other of the contracted holds that may be more difficult to perform.

STARTING POSITION

Sit on your heels with your hands on your knees, your back straight, and your head in line with your spine.

INITIAL INHALATION

In four counts, stretch your arms above your head, opening your shoulders and your chest well while inhaling directly, completely, and calmly.

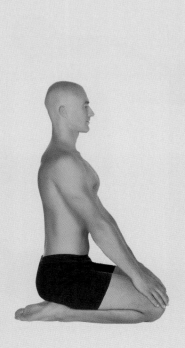

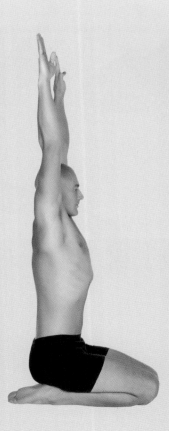

INITIAL EXHALATION

Exhaling directly and fully in four counts, bend forward with your spine and arms stretched and controlled to place your palms on the floor. Curl your toes under and, for a moment, suspend your body in a straight line on your toes and palms, with your arms straight and perpendicular to the floor.

When stretching forward, your palms should be placed to be at the level of your shoulders, as in the Snake Yantra.

CENTRAL INHALATION

Without pausing, inhale directly and forcefully in two counts and arch your head and torso back while remaining suspended on your hands and toes.

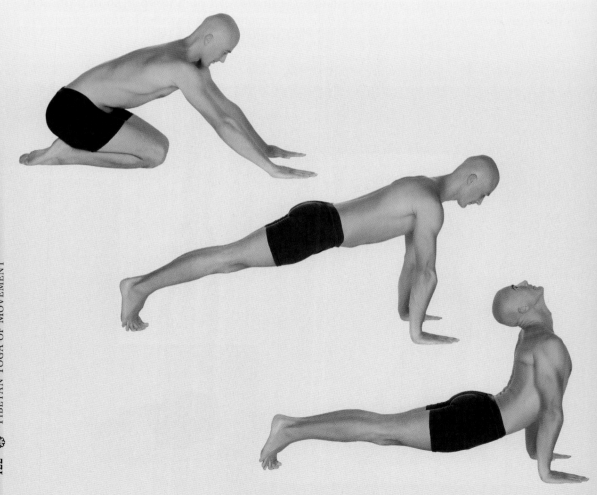

CONTRACTED HOLD

Interrupting your breathing by forcefully emitting an aspirated "HA," quickly bring your head between your straight arms while raising your buttocks up and back to form a right angle with your legs and arms. Your head, back, and arms are in a straight line. Keep your heels and the soles of your feet firmly on the floor and your legs thoroughly stretched.

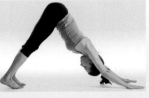

If you cannot keep your feet flat on the floor, try to gently press your heels toward the floor as much as possible without bending your knees.

Then stay in contracted hold for six counts, pulling your abdominal muscles in as you gently pull your pelvis back, remaining in this position like a stretching dog, with your arms and legs actively extended throughout the hold.

CENTRAL EXHALATION

In two counts, exhale quickly yet fully and lie down with your toes curled under and your hands alongside your chest. Then remain empty for two counts.

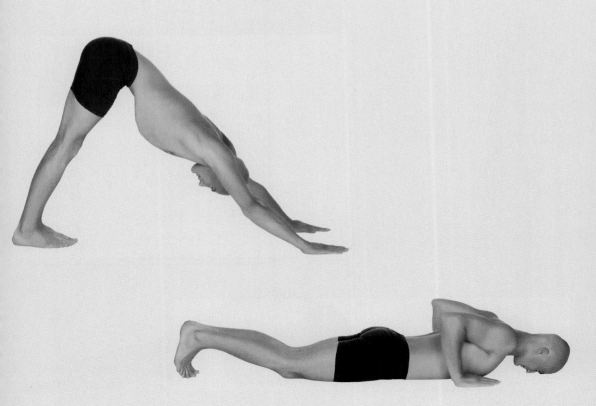

CONCLUDING INHALATION

In four counts, inhaling directly and fully, place the tops of your feet on the floor and come up to sit on your heels with your arms well extended and parallel alongside your head.

CONCLUDING EXHALATION

In four counts, exhale calmly as you bend forward to bring your forehead to the floor and your arms straight in front of you.

REPETITION

To enjoy the full potential of the benefits of this Yantra, repeat the entire sequence two more times, either returning to the starting position while continuing to inhale and exhale calmly, or linking the final exhalation directly to the initial inhalation of the next round.

TRANSITION

To link the Dog to the starting position for the next Yantra, the Spider, inhale, coming up to sit on your heels with your toes curled under and your arms raised over your head. Exhale, rolling back to sit on your buttocks while stretching your legs forward and placing your hands on your knees.

HEALTH BENEFITS

- *Alleviates complaints related to the spine and spinal cord*
- *Improves the condition of the ligaments and tendons*
- *Relieves disorders of the kidneys*
- *Alleviates ailments of the small and large intestines*
- *Eases heartburn, abdominal bloating, and poor or difficult digestion*
- *Counteracts problems caused by the damaged or disordered functioning of the pervasive prana*

Related Warm-Ups (see Appendix 1): Snake Training (33), Snake Training II (34), Dog Training (36)

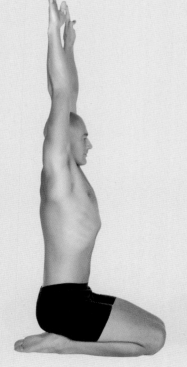

BREATHING CYCLE		COUNTS
Initial Inhalation		4
Initial Exhalation		4
Central Inhalation		2
Contracted Hold		**6**
Central Exhalation	Exhalation	2
	Empty Hold	2
Concluding Inhalation		4
Concluding Exhalation		4

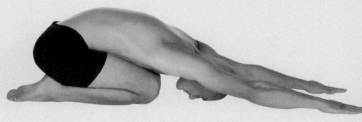

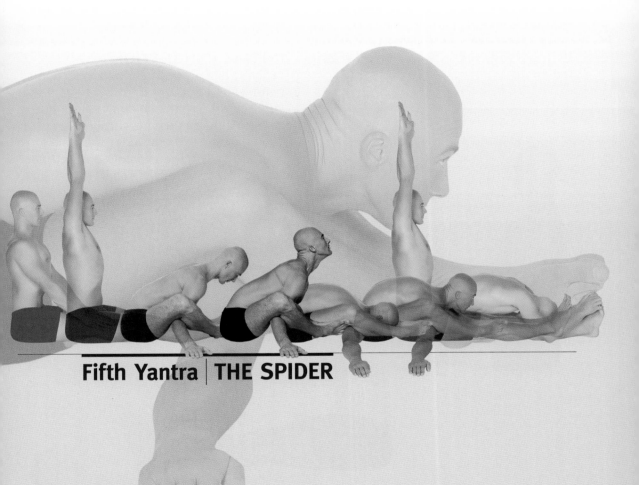

Fifth Yantra | **THE SPIDER**

THE SPIDER IS for experiencing and training empty hold. In the central phase, we exhale forcefully in two counts and then remain empty for six counts. All other cycles are done in four counts.

STARTING POSITION

Sit with your legs in front of you and your hands on your knees, present and alert with your back straight and in alignment. Your breathing is relaxed and calm.

A support like a thin cushion under your buttocks may make it easier to perform the Spider.

INITIAL INHALATION

In four counts, extend your arms over your head as you open and expand your chest and your shoulders, keeping your arms straight alongside your head.

INITIAL EXHALATION

Exhaling directly and calmly in four counts, bend your legs, open your knees wide apart, and bring the soles of your feet together. At the same time, slowly lower your arms and pass them under the backs of your knees with your palms on the floor, spreading your arms wide apart to the sides as you lower your torso straight forward.

CENTRAL INHALATION

In four counts, inhale directly and calmly while arching your chest and head upward and stretching your abdomen, with your knees bearing down on your arms.

CENTRAL EXHALATION

In two counts, quickly and strongly exhale, lowering your chest and head to the floor while sliding your buttocks backward.

One way to help you slide back in this phase is to do this Yantra on a smooth surface like a wooden floor instead of on a mat. Nevertheless, sliding may not be easy for everyone, but not doing it will not hamper the effectiveness of the Yantra.

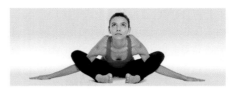

It is also possible to keep the feet slightly apart if it makes the position easier.

EMPTY HOLD

Holding empty for six counts, arch your head upward and back, and remain in this pose, which resembles a spider.

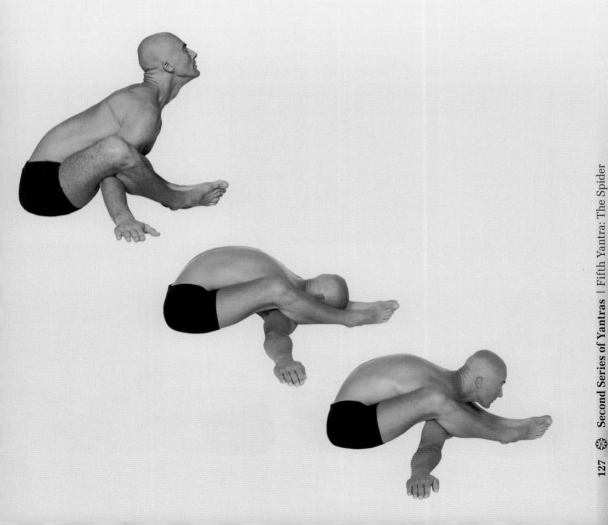

CONCLUDING INHALATION

Inhaling fully in four counts, expand your chest well as you extend your arms over your head and stretch your legs forward.

CONCLUDING EXHALATION

Exhaling in four counts, bend forward from the base of your spine, bringing your forehead to your knees and your fingers to your toes.

As already explained, work with your condition and capacity. Do not force anything. If you cannot bring your forehead to your knees and your fingers to your toes, just remember to release your spine from *pressure, moving gently from the base, and stop wherever you feel comfortable.*

REPETITION

To enjoy the full potential of the benefits of this Yantra, repeat the entire sequence two more times, either returning to the starting position while continuing to inhale and exhale calmly, or linking the final exhalation directly to the initial inhalation of the next round.

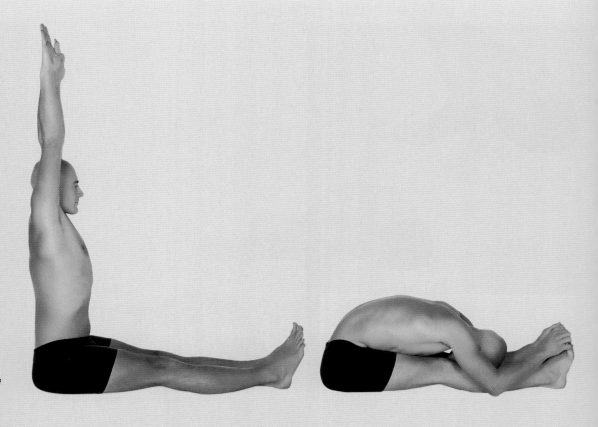

TRANSITION

If you are doing the second and third series in a single session, you can link the Spider to the first Yantra of the third series, the Bow, by inhaling as you raise your arms over your head, then exhaling as you bring your heels toward your perineum, lower your arms, and roll forward onto your knees to sit on your heels with the tops of your feet flat on the floor and your hands resting on your knees.

HEALTH BENEFITS

- *Benefits the five solid organs in general*
- *Relieves ailments of the heart and kidneys*
- *Eases pain in the lumbar region*
- *Alleviates disorders of a cold nature*
- *Improves poor digestion*
- *Eases pain in the upper torso accompanied by a sensation of swelling resulting from high blood pressure*
- *Dissolves calculi*
- *Restores the balance of all five pranas when their functioning is damaged or disordered*

Related Warm-Ups (see Appendix 1): Rotating the Legs (6), Butterfly (8), Both Knees to the Side Forward Bend (13), Turning and Stretching (15)

BREATHING CYCLE	COUNTS
Initial Inhalation	4
Initial Exhalation	4
Central Inhalation	4
Central Exhalation	2
Empty Hold	**6**
Concluding Inhalation	4
Concluding Exhalation	4

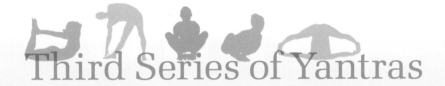

Third Series of Yantras

THE FIVE YANTRAS in the third series are the Bow for open hold, the Half-Moon for directed hold, the Lion for closed hold, the Vulture for contracted hold, and the Triangle for empty hold. This series includes the only Yantra of all twenty-five that is a standing position, the Half-Moon. The third series as a whole helps train and deepen the function of closed hold in particular.

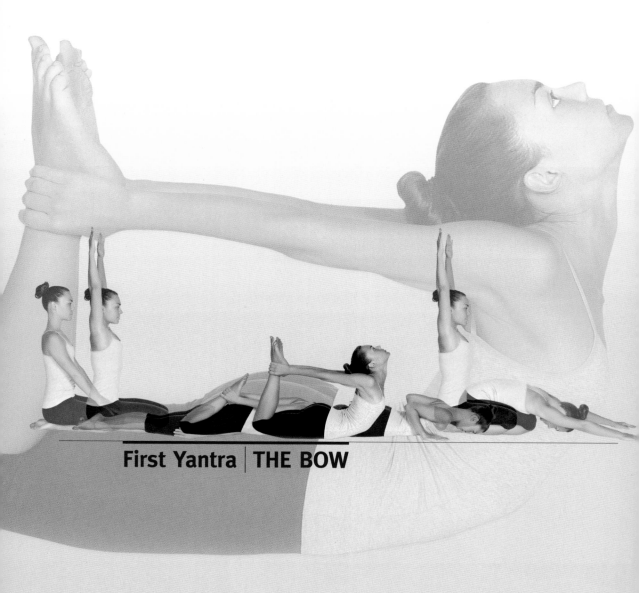

First Yantra | **THE BOW**

THE BOW IS for applying, experiencing, and training open hold. All seven breathing cycles are done to a count of four, consciously coordinating the movement and breath with the rhythm while breathing directly, completely, and calmly. Always strive to be present, alert, and yet relaxed, doing all movements with calm intent.

STARTING POSITION
Sit on your heels with your back straight and your hands on your knees. Your breathing is relaxed and natural.

INITIAL INHALATION
Inhaling directly, completely, and calmly in four counts, extend your arms straight over your head and open your shoulders and your chest well to facilitate a full expansion of the breath.

INITIAL EXHALATION
Exhaling calmly for four counts, reach your arms in front of you and place your palms on the floor to come into a prone position with your arms along your sides and your forehead on the floor.

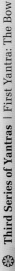

CENTRAL INHALATION

Inhaling completely, slowly, and directly for four counts, reach back with your hands to firmly grasp your ankles, placing your thumbs on the inside.

OPEN HOLD

Holding open for four counts, stretch your arms and legs strongly as you pull your feet up and away from your body without raising your knees. At the same time as arching your head back, raise your torso and push your chest out, forming a shape like a bow.

Hold on to your ankles strongly and push your knees to or toward the floor while opening your chest and allowing your held air to keep expanding. Strive to keep your

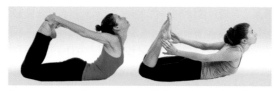

knees together or parallel and on the floor.

To make the position easier, you can keep your knees slightly above the floor or separate them a little. You can also grab your feet instead of your ankles, or simply reach as close to your feet as possible.

CENTRAL EXHALATION

Exhaling directly and calmly in four counts, lower your legs and chest and place your forehead on the floor and your palms at chest level.

You can also place your hands a bit farther back to make the next movement smoother and easier.

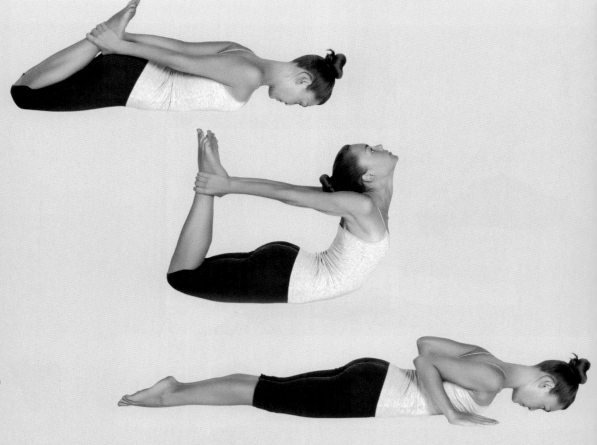

CONCLUDING INHALATION

Inhaling deeply in four counts, come up to sit on your heels as you raise your arms over your head and open your chest.

CONCLUDING EXHALATION

Exhaling in four counts, lower your forehead to the floor in front of your knees and reach your arms forward, placing your palms on the floor without lifting your buttocks off your heels.

REPETITION

To enjoy the full potential of the benefits of this Yantra, repeat the entire sequence two more times, either returning to the starting position while continuing to inhale and exhale calmly, or linking the final exhalation directly to the initial inhalation of the next round.

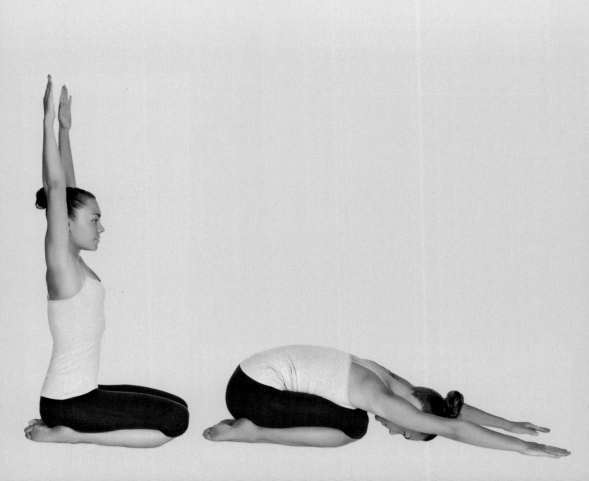

TRANSITION

To link the Bow in a sequence to the starting position for the next Yantra, the Half-Moon, inhale fully and directly as you curl your toes under and come up into a standing position with your arms raised above your head. Then exhale as you lower your arms along your sides, keeping your legs straight and parallel with your knees relaxed and your back straight.

HEALTH BENEFITS

- *Relieves ailments of the spine and spinal cord*
- *Alleviates disorders of the kidneys*
- *Eases pain in the joints and bones of the lumbar region*
- *Alleviates problems of the ligaments and tendons of the torso and limbs*
- *Improves appetite and digestion*
- *Relieves ailments of the five solid and six hollow organs*
- *Counteracts problems caused by damaged, impaired, or disordered functioning of the five pranas*

Related Warm-Ups (see Appendix 1): Bridge (29), Cat (31), Locust Training (32), Snake Training (33), Snake Training II (34), Neck Roll (37), Shoulder and Chest Opener (39)

BREATHING CYCLE	COUNTS
Initial Inhalation	4
Initial Exhalation	4
Central Inhalation	4
Open Hold	**4**
Central Exhalation	4
Concluding Inhalation	4
Concluding Exhalation	4

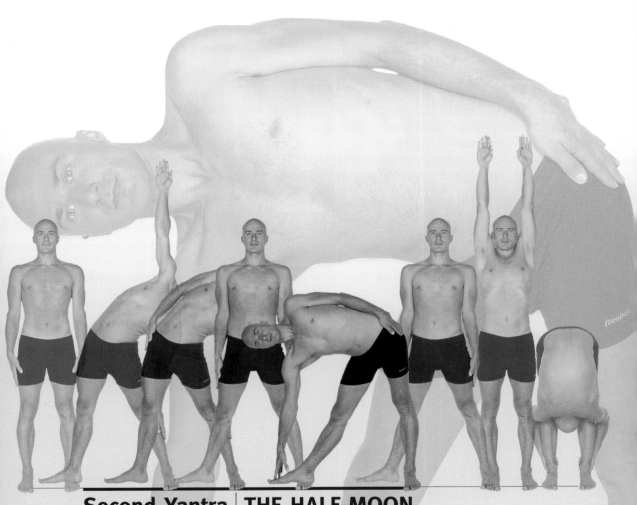

Second Yantra | THE HALF-MOON

137

THE HALF-MOON IS for applying, experiencing, and training directed hold. All seven breathing cycles are done in four counts, breathing directly, completely, and calmly. As an asymmetrical sequence, men and women start on opposite sides.

STARTING POSITION
Stand with your arms at your sides, your legs and feet parallel, relaxed but alert, with your spine correctly aligned.

INITIAL INHALATION
Inhaling in four counts, turn one foot out to the side as you step out two hand spans to the same side with your leg while tensing your whole body and extending the corresponding arm up, keeping your gaze fixed on the fingers of the elevated hand. At the same time, bend your torso to the other side and firmly press your hand on that side down along your thigh to below the knee for a massaging effect.

In the first round, women turn the left foot out while stepping out to the side with the left leg, raising the left arm up, and pressing the right hand down along the right leg. Men turn the right foot out while stepping out to the side with the right leg, raising the right arm up, and pressing the left hand down along the left leg.

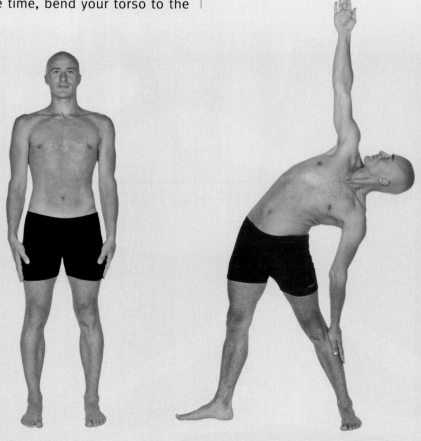

Open your leg about two hand spans out to the side (or more, to make the position easier), placing your extended foot at a perpendicular angle to your other foot, which remains firmly pointing forward. It is important not to turn the pelvis while bending to the side.

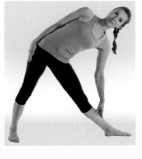

INITIAL EXHALATION

Exhaling directly and calmly in four counts, slowly lower your raised arm to your side without releasing the position of your other hand.

CENTRAL INHALATION

Inhaling directly and calmly in four counts, slowly straighten your torso, tensing your whole body while massaging your thighs by pulling your lower palm up and pressing your other palm downward.

DIRECTED HOLD

Applying a directed hold for four counts, bend your torso toward your extended foot without turning your hips and slide your fingers as far as your toes, forming a half-moon shape with your body.

In the first round, women bend the torso to the left, bringing the fingers to the toes of the left foot; men bend to the right and bring the fingers to the toes of the right foot.

To allow the full experience of the directed hold, do not bring your fingers toward your toes too slowly. Enough time should remain so you can pause in the Half-Moon position. If you cannot reach your toes, simply go as far as you can.

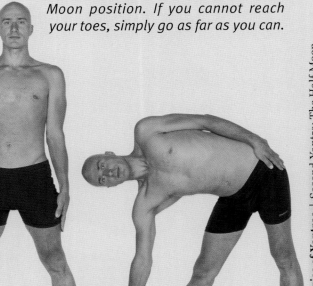

CENTRAL EXHALATION

Exhaling directly and calmly in four counts, slowly rise back up to a vertical position, leaving your arms along your sides and keeping your legs apart.

CONCLUDING INHALATION

Inhaling directly and calmly in four counts, extend your arms over your head, expanding your chest and bringing your feet parallel and slightly apart to keep a firm balance.

CONCLUDING EXHALATION

Exhaling directly and calmly in four counts, bend forward from the root of your spine in a controlled but relaxed manner, grab your ankles, and bring your forehead to your knees.

When you wrap your hands around your ankles, keep the thumbs in front.

REPETITION

Repeat the entire sequence on the opposite side, either returning to the starting position while continuing to inhale and exhale calmly, or linking the final exhalation directly to the initial inhalation of the second round. Then continue as before, but reversing the position of your arms and legs.

In the second round, women turn the right foot out while stepping the right leg out to the side, raising the right arm up, and pressing the left hand down along the left leg. Men turn the left foot out while stepping the left leg out to the side, raising the left arm up, and pressing the right hand down along the right leg.

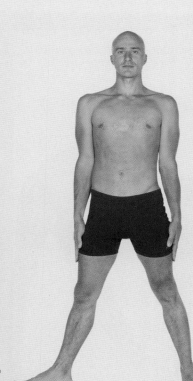
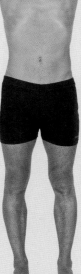
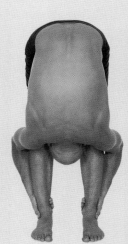

TRANSITION

To link the Half-Moon in a sequence to the starting position for the next Yantra in the third series, the Lion, inhale fully and directly as you sit down on your buttocks while extending your arms over your head and joining the soles of your feet together, not too close to your body. Then exhale calmly and directly, bringing your hands to your knees and keeping your back straight.

You can first put your hands on the floor at your sides to help you sit back on your buttocks.

BREATHING CYCLE	COUNTS
Initial Inhalation	4
Initial Exhalation	4
Central Inhalation	4
Directed Hold	**4**
Central Exhalation	4
Concluding Inhalation	4
Concluding Exhalation	4

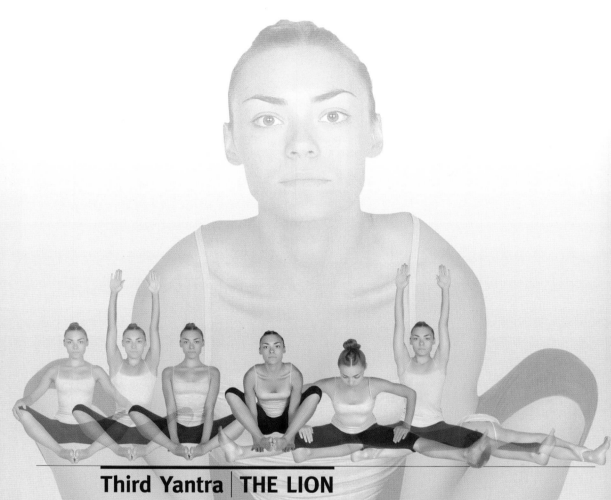

Third Yantra | THE LION

THE LION IS for applying, experiencing, and training closed hold. In the central phase, a two-count inhalation is followed by a six-count closed hold. All other cycles are done in four counts, breathing directly, completely, and calmly.

STARTING POSITION

Sit with the soles of your feet together, not too close to your perineum, with your hands on your open knees and your back straight.

You may find it helpful to place a thin cushion or firm prop under your buttocks for this Yantra.

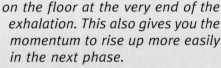

INITIAL INHALATION

Inhaling directly in four counts, stretch your arms up and open your chest to facilitate a full inhalation.

INITIAL EXHALATION

Exhaling in four counts, bring your hands in front of your perineum, either with your fingers forward and your palms on the floor or in vajra fists.

Synchronize the downward movement of your hands so that you arrive to place them on the floor at the very end of the exhalation. This also gives you the momentum to rise up more easily in the next phase.

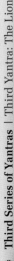

CENTRAL INHALATION

Inhaling quickly and directly in two counts, straighten your arms and back and open your shoulders as you lift your buttocks and feet off the floor, supporting yourself on your hands.

If you cannot lift your feet off the floor, raise only your buttocks. If that is also not possible, stay seated on the floor, making sure to open your chest and stretch your arms and torso well.

CLOSED HOLD

For six counts, hold closed in this position, which resembles a lion, keeping your back straight and your chest open and tensing your whole body. Still holding the air, start coming back to the floor on the fifth count. The dynamics of the position convey a clear experience of closed hold, with the sides thoroughly tightened and the air firmly blocked down below the navel.

CENTRAL EXHALATION

Exhaling fully and calmly in four counts, extend your legs apart, place your hands on your knees with the thumbs on the outside, and bend forward a little to finish expelling the air.

Bend forward only as far as is comfortable.

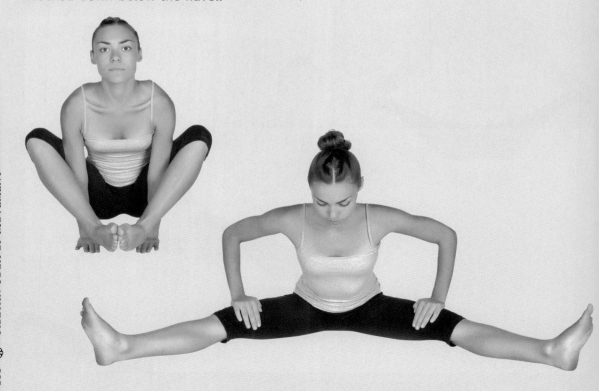

CONCLUDING INHALATION

Inhaling calmly in four counts, stretch your arms up, expanding your chest.

CONCLUDING EXHALATION

Exhaling calmly in four counts, bend forward to place your forearms on your extended legs. Bring your forehead to or toward the floor, keeping your back straight.

Again, bend forward only as far as is comfortable.

REPETITION

To enjoy the full potential of the benefits of this Yantra, repeat the entire sequence two more times, either returning to the starting position while continuing to inhale and exhale calmly, or linking the final exhalation directly to the initial inhalation of the next round.

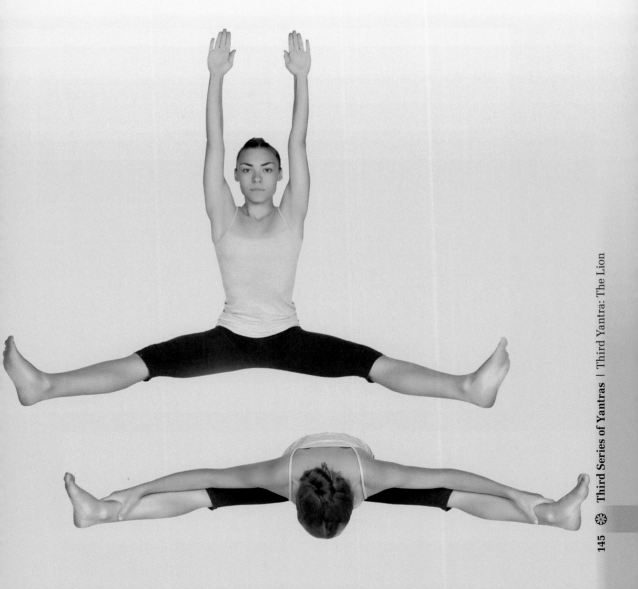

TRANSITION

To link the Lion in a sequence to the next Yantra in the third series, the Vulture, inhale, raising your arms up parallel over your head, then exhale, bringing the soles of your feet together in front of your perineum with your hands on your knees in *tsokyil* position.

HEALTH BENEFITS

- *Alleviates ailments of the spine and spinal cord*
- *Improves the condition of the major and minor joints*
- *Relieves disorders related to the ligaments of the head and limbs*
- *Alleviates ailments of the five solid and six hollow organs*
- *Counteracts problems caused by the impaired functioning of the five pranas*

Related Warm-Ups (see Appendix 1): Snake Training (33), Snake Training II (34), Neck Roll (37)

BREATHING CYCLE	COUNTS
Initial Inhalation	4
Initial Exhalation	4
Central Inhalation	2
Closed Hold	**6**
Central Exhalation	4
Concluding Inhalation	4
Concluding Exhalation	4

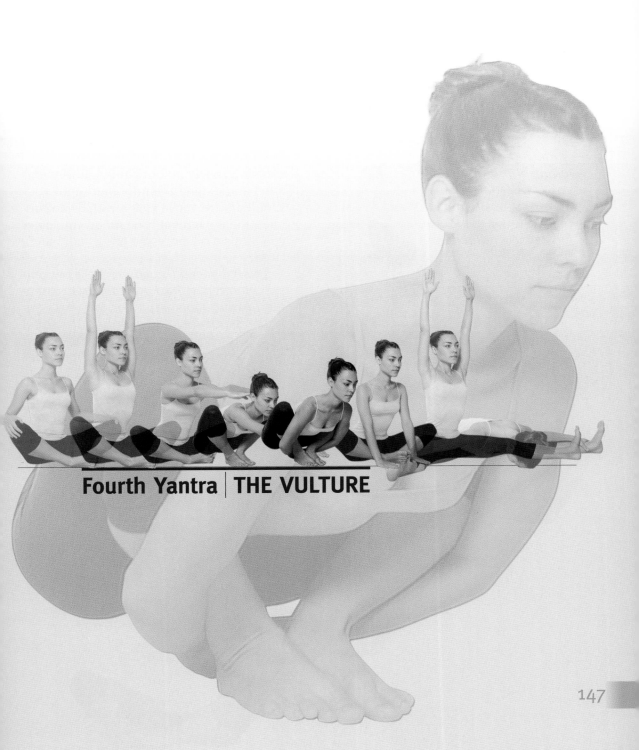

Fourth Yantra | THE VULTURE

THE VULTURE IS for applying, experiencing, and training contracted hold. All seven breathing cycles are done to a count of four. Although it is a symmetrical pose, women and men clasp the opposite hand behind the back in the central phase.

STARTING POSITION

Sit with the soles of your feet together, knees wide apart, and your hands on your knees, relaxed and yet attentive.

Placing a thin cushion or firm prop under your buttocks may make this position and the following movements easier and more precise.

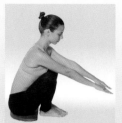

INITIAL INHALATION

Inhaling calmly in four counts, raise your arms up and expand your chest well.

INITIAL EXHALATION

Exhaling calmly in four counts, lower your arms and extend them forward until your shoulders are above your knees. Then continue the movement forward as you lower your arms a bit more and bring your hands closer.

This movement needs to be slow and synchronized with your breathing to create the forward momentum for the next step in the sequence. You may find it helpful to add a little bounce to your movement to get yourself up. Alternatively, use your hands to push yourself off the floor. In that case, time the push at the end of the exhalation to avoid blocking and tensing your breathing.

CENTRAL INHALATION

Inhaling calmly in four counts, push your arms and torso forward and use the momentum to come up onto your feet by placing the soles of your feet on the floor. Then lift your buttocks while wrapping your arms around your open knees, making a vajra fist with one hand, and grabbing hold of your wrist with the other hand just above your heels, thus entering what is called the position of the yogin.

Women make a vajra fist with the left hand and grab the left wrist with the right hand; men make a vajra fist with the right hand and grab the right wrist with the left hand. The placement of the hands does not alternate in subsequent rounds.

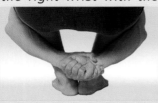

If you cannot wrap your hand around your wrist, you can just link your fingers. Alternatively, bring your hands as close together behind your back as possible or reach them back along the sides.

CONTRACTED HOLD

Planting your heels firmly on the floor, apply contracted hold for four counts while energetically arching your head and your torso back, remaining suspended in this squatting pose, which resembles a vulture.

To fully experience the contracted hold, pull your abdomen back toward your spine. If you cannot keep your heels firmly on the floor, you can take the position with your heels partly raised.

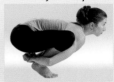

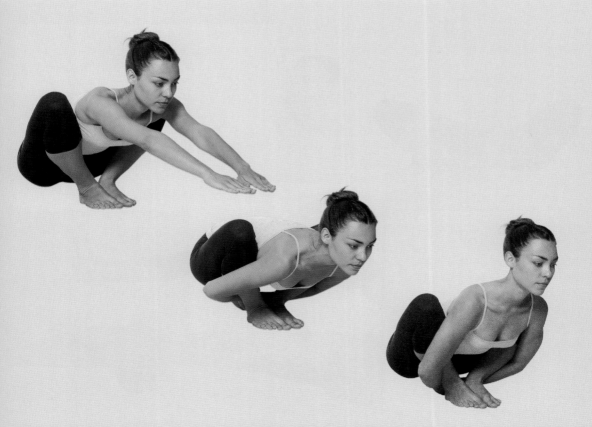

CENTRAL EXHALATION

Completely and calmly exhaling in four counts, sit back on the floor with the soles of your feet together and your shoulders open, bringing your hands beside your feet and keeping your arms and your back straight.

CONCLUDING INHALATION

Inhale calmly in four counts, extending your legs wide apart and raising your arms up.

CONCLUDING EXHALATION

Exhale calmly and fully in four counts, bringing your forehead to or toward the floor while keeping your back straight and placing your forearms on your extended legs.

Bend forward only as far as is comfortable.

REPETITION

To enjoy the full potential of the benefits of this Yantra, repeat the entire sequence two more times, either returning to the starting position while continuing to inhale and exhale calmly, or linking the final exhalation directly to the initial inhalation of the next round.

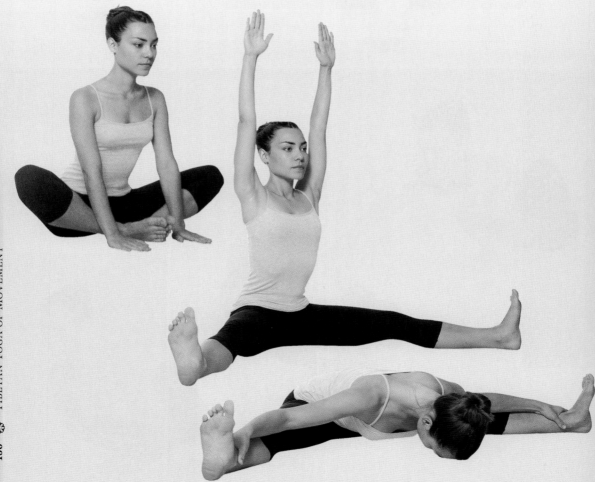

TRANSITION

To link the Vulture in a sequence to the next Yantra in the third series, the Triangle, inhale, straightening your back and raising your arms up alongside your head. Exhale, bringing the soles of your feet together in front of your perineum and your hands to your knees.

HEALTH BENEFITS

- *Balances the functioning of the five pranas and the five elements*
- *Counteracts problems caused by the damaged or abnormal functioning of the ascending prana*
- *Restores and tonifies the nerves connected with the five solid organs and with the five sense organs*

Related Warm-Ups (see Appendix 1): Squat (3), Butterfly (8), Transition Training (22), Soles Together Hip Opener (35)

Breathing Cycle	Counts
Initial Inhalation	4
Initial Exhalation	4
Central Inhalation	4
Contracted Hold	**4**
Central Exhalation	4
Concluding Inhalation	4
Concluding Exhalation	4

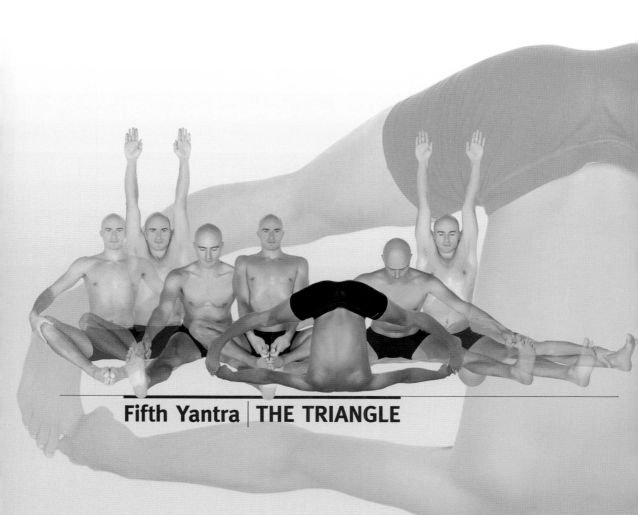

Fifth Yantra | THE TRIANGLE

THE TRIANGLE IS for applying, experiencing, and training empty hold. The empty hold lasts six counts and follows a two-count exhalation. All other cycles are done in four counts, breathing directly, completely, and calmly.

STARTING POSITION
Sit with the soles of your feet together, knees wide apart, and your hands on your knees, relaxed and present.

INITIAL INHALATION
In four counts, inhale calmly and fully, extending your arms straight up to expand the chest well.

INITIAL EXHALATION
Exhaling calmly and fully in four counts, stretch your legs forward, opening them apart at a narrow angle. At the same time, lower your arms and close your hands in vajra fists, leaving your index fingers free and hooking them around your big toes.

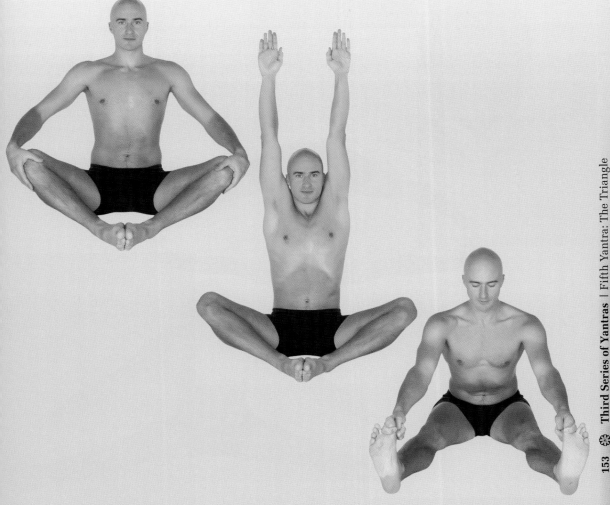

CENTRAL INHALATION

Inhaling calmly and fully in four counts, slowly pull your heels to the perineum while straightening your back and expanding your chest.

CENTRAL EXHALATION

Exhaling quickly and completely in two counts, roll back while straightening your legs and arms, with your fingers still hooked around your big toes, and bring your feet to the floor with your legs wide apart.

To make it easier and softer to move into this position, you can place a small mat or thick blanket at the mid-cervical region. Your head should be placed off the mat and on the floor. Do not force yourself into this position if you do not feel comfortable with it.

EMPTY HOLD

Hold empty for six counts, keeping the back of your head, your shoulders, and your toes on the floor and forming the shape of a triangle. At the end of the fifth count, vigorously roll forward, bringing your extended legs to the floor in front while keeping them wide open.

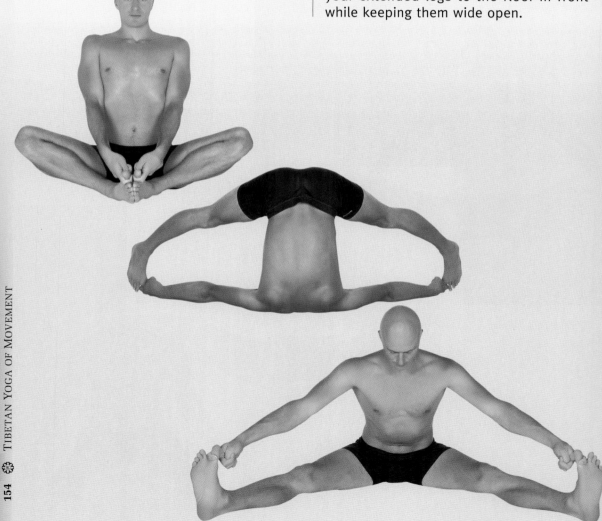

Keep your legs thoroughly tense to avoid hitting the floor with your heels. To make it easier, you may want to join your feet at first to help you roll forward, and then open your legs apart at the end of the forward movement.

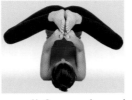

CONCLUDING INHALATION

Inhaling calmly and fully in four counts, raise your arms above your head and open your chest.

CONCLUDING EXHALATION

Exhaling calmly and fully in four counts, bend forward and lower your forehead to the floor while bringing your forearms to your extended legs.

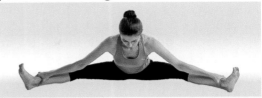

If you cannot bring your forehead to the ground, simply bend as far as possible without forcing, keeping your back straight. As in the previous Yantras, maintain awareness of the alignment of your spine as you bend forward, going only as far as is comfortable, even if it means simply remaining seated and placing your hands on your knees at the end of the exhalation.

REPETITION

To enjoy the full potential of the benefits of this Yantra, repeat the entire sequence two more times, either returning to the starting position while continuing to inhale and exhale calmly, or linking the final exhalation directly to the initial inhalation of the next round.

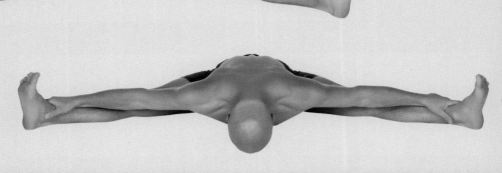

TRANSITION

If you are doing the third and fourth series in a single session, you can link the Triangle to the first Yantra of the fourth series, the Locust. Inhale directly and slowly as you raise your arms over your head while joining your legs straight in front. Exhale slowly and directly, bringing your heels toward your perineum while lowering your arms and rolling forward onto your knees to sit on your heels with the tops of your feet flat on the floor and your hands resting on your knees.

HEALTH BENEFITS

- *Alleviates disorders of the spine and spinal cord*
- *Relieves ailments of the five solid and six hollow organs*
- *Improves conditions related to the muscles, ligaments, and tendons of the head and limbs*
- *Counteracts problems caused by damaged or impaired functioning of the five pranas by harmonizing and strengthening them*

Related Warm-Ups (see Appendix 1): Turning and Stretching (15), Side Stretch (19), Open Forward Stretch (20), Spine Roll (30)

BREATHING CYCLE	COUNTS
Initial Inhalation	4
Initial Exhalation	4
Central Inhalation	4
Central Exhalation	2
Empty Hold	**6**
Concluding Inhalation	4
Concluding Exhalation	4

Fourth Series of Yantras

THE FIVE YANTRAS in the fourth series are the Locust for open hold, the Dove for directed hold, the Trident for closed hold, the Tiger for contracted hold, and the Jewel for empty hold. In this series, when we finish the sequence of the last three Yantras with a forward bending exhalation, we grab the sides of the feet instead of joining fingers with the toes. The fourth series as a whole helps train and deepen the function of contracted hold in particular.

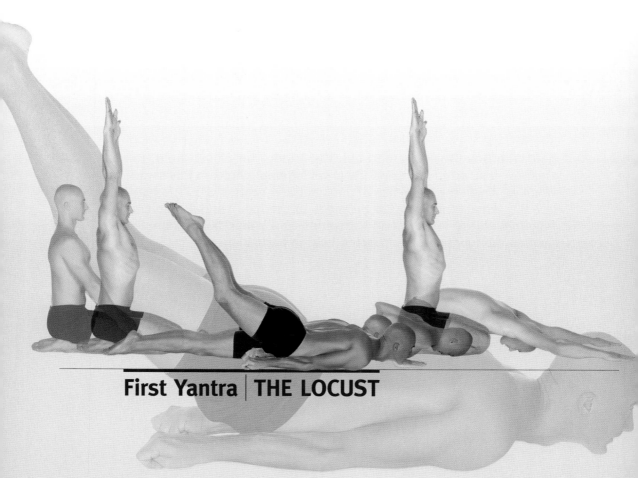

First Yantra | **THE LOCUST**

THE LOCUST IS for applying, experiencing, and training open hold. All seven breathing cycles are done to a count of four, breathing directly, fully, and calmly through the nose.

STARTING POSITION

Sit on your heels with your hands on your knees and your back straight, relaxed yet attentive and present.

INITIAL INHALATION

Inhaling calmly and fully in four counts, stretch your arms straight up, expanding your chest well.

INITIAL EXHALATION

Exhaling calmly and fully in four counts, lie down in a prone position with your forehead on the floor, arms along your sides, and hands in vajra fists.

To make the movement easier, you can place the vajra fists or even the palms of your hands slightly under your thighs toward the end of the exhalation.

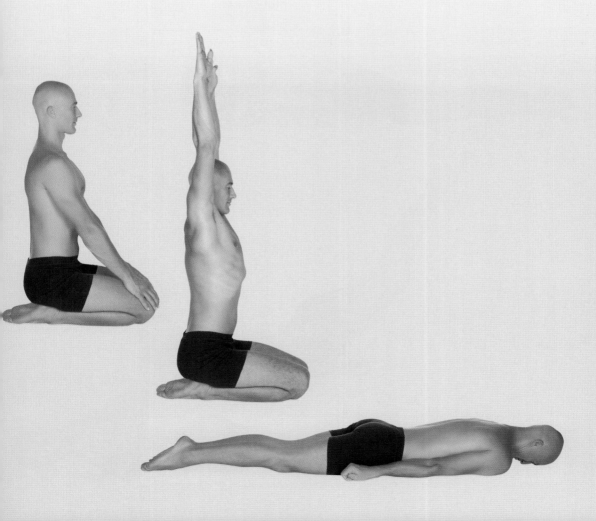

CENTRAL INHALATION

Inhaling calmly and fully from the bottom up in four counts, roll your head back to rest your chin and throat on the floor. At the same time, vigorously stretch through your legs while tensing your whole body.

OPEN HOLD

Holding open for four counts, lift your extended legs and your pelvis as high off the floor as you can. Support the weight of your body on your shoulders and arms with your fists or hands firmly pressed on the floor. Hold the lower part of your body arched upward like a locust for the remainder of the count.

Keep your legs close together and controlled. It is not important how high you manage to lift your body off the floor. Go only as far as your capacity allows, making sure that the held air is not blocked. For beginners it may be easier to bend the legs a little while attempting to keep the knees and feet as close together as possible.

CENTRAL EXHALATION

Exhaling calmly and fully in four counts, bring your legs down, placing your forehead on the floor and your palms at chest level or lower.

If you place your hands lower than chest level, it will be easier to perform the next movement.

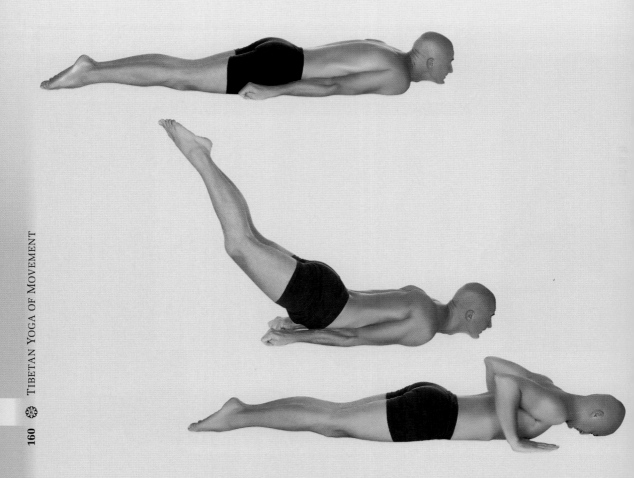

CONCLUDING INHALATION

Inhaling calmly and fully in four counts, come up to sit on your heels and stretch your arms up to expand your chest well and straighten your spine.

CONCLUDING EXHALATION

Exhaling in four counts, bring your forehead and your palms to the floor as you expel the air completely and calmly.

REPETITION

To enjoy the full potential of the benefits of this Yantra, repeat the entire sequence two more times, either returning to the starting position while continuing to inhale and exhale calmly, or linking the final exhalation directly to the initial inhalation of the next round.

TRANSITION

To link the Locust to the next Yantra in the fourth series, the Dove, inhale, rising back up from the concluding exhalation and stretching your arms over your head. Then exhale and place your hands on your knees.

HEALTH BENEFITS

- *Alleviates ailments of the spine and spinal cord*
- *Improves the condition of the major and minor joints*
- *Relieves disorders related to the ligaments of the head and limbs*
- *Alleviates ailments of the five solid and six hollow organs*
- *Counteracts problems caused by the impaired functioning of the five pranas*

Related Warm-Ups (see Appendix 1): Snake Training (33), Snake Training II (34), Neck Roll (37)

BREATHING CYCLE	COUNTS
Initial Inhalation	4
Initial Exhalation	4
Central Inhalation	4
Open Hold	**4**
Central Exhalation	4
Concluding Inhalation	4
Concluding Exhalation	4

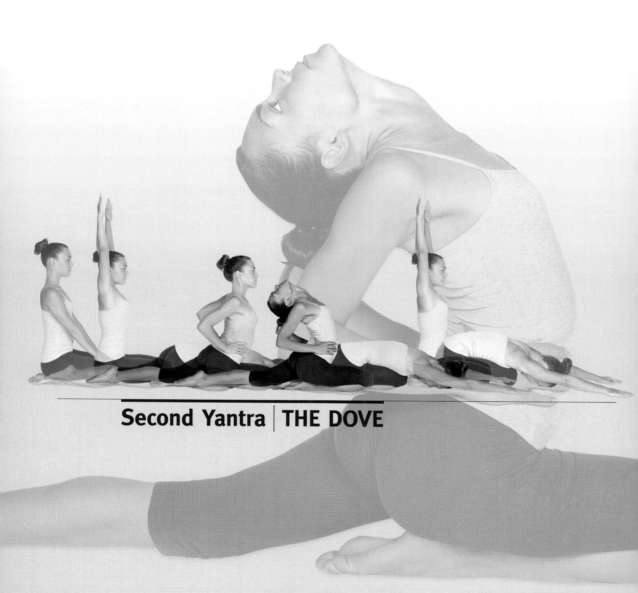

Second Yantra | THE DOVE

THE DOVE IS for applying, experiencing, and training directed hold. All seven breathing cycles are done to a count of four, breathing directly, fully, and calmly through the nose.

STARTING POSITION

Sit on your heels with your hands on your knees. Your arms are straight and you are relaxed yet present.

INITIAL INHALATION

Inhaling fully and calmly in four counts, stretch your arms up alongside your head, straightening and aligning your back and opening and expanding your chest.

INITIAL EXHALATION

Exhaling fully and calmly in four counts, stretch your arms and torso forward and bring your palms and your forehead to the floor as you extend one leg straight back, leaving the other leg bent with heel pressed to or toward your perineum.

In the first round, women extend the left leg back and men extend the right leg back.

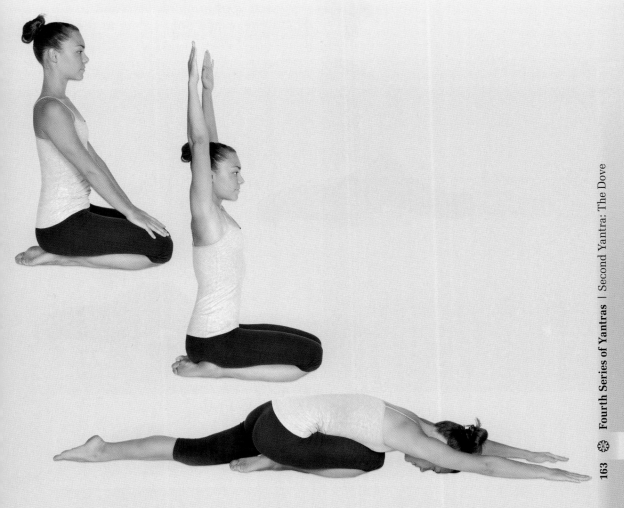

CENTRAL INHALATION

Inhaling fully and calmly in four counts, raise your torso up and bring your hands to your sides below your ribs with the fingers in front and the thumbs behind, pulling your elbows back and arching your spine to open your chest and shoulders well.

You can also first slide your hands back along the sides of the thigh of your bent leg to help you come up into the arching position more easily.

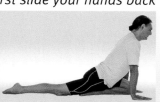

DIRECTED HOLD

Apply directed hold for four counts as you arch your head farther back, push your chest farther out, keep pulling your elbows toward each other, and firmly press your perineum to your heel, remaining in this position, which resembles the shape of a dove.

The dynamics of the position allow the held air to be directed toward the lower abdomen. Pressing your heel toward your perineum helps you fully experience the function of this Yantra.

CENTRAL EXHALATION

Exhaling fully and calmly in four counts, reach your arms forward and bring your forehead and your palms to the floor in front of you.

CONCLUDING INHALATION

Inhaling fully and calmly in four counts, raise your torso up as you bring your extended leg forward to sit on your heels in a kneeling position while raising your arms up to align your spine.

As in the central inhalation cycle, you can first slide your hands forward along the sides of the thigh of your bent leg to make it easier to come to sit on your heels.

CONCLUDING EXHALATION

Exhaling fully and calmly in four counts, stretch your arms out straight as you bend forward and bring your forehead and your palms to the floor in front of you.

REPETITION

Repeat the entire sequence on the opposite side, either returning to the starting position while continuing to inhale and exhale calmly, or linking the final exhalation directly to the initial inhalation of the second round. Then continue as before, but reversing the position of your arms and legs.

In the second round, women extend the right leg back and men extend the left leg back.

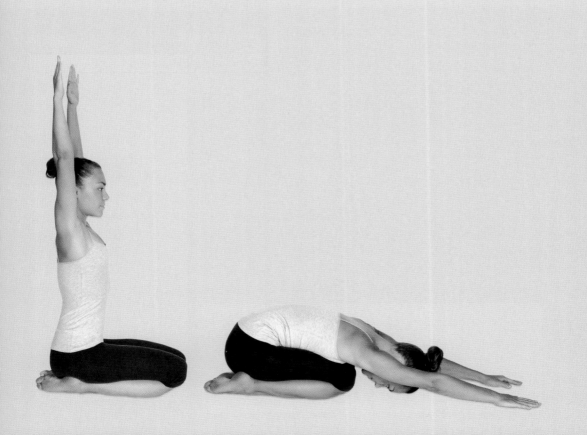

TRANSITION

To link the Dove in a sequence to the starting position for the next Yantra, the Trident, inhale, coming up to sit on your heels with your toes curled under and your arms raised over your head. Exhale, rolling back to sit on your buttocks while stretching your legs forward and placing your hands on your knees.

HEALTH BENEFITS

- *Alleviates ailments of the upper torso*
- *Eases shoulder pain*
- *Improves conditions related to imbalances of phlegm energy in general*
- *Relieves gastritis and heartburn*
- *Counteracts problems caused by the disordered or impaired functioning of the ascending and pervasive pranas*

Related Warm-Ups (see Appendix 1): Knees to the Chest (9), Turning and Stretching (15), Knee Bend (16), Gentle Spine Twist (21), Snake Training (33), Snake Training II (34), Neck Roll (37)

BREATHING CYCLE	COUNTS
Initial Inhalation	4
Initial Exhalation	4
Central Inhalation	4
Directed Hold	**4**
Central Exhalation	4
Concluding Inhalation	4
Concluding Exhalation	4

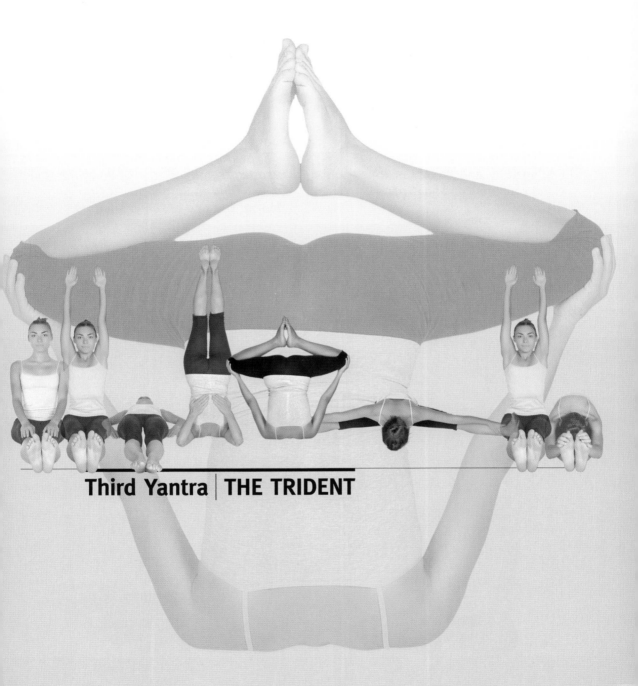

Third Yantra | **THE TRIDENT**

THE TRIDENT IS for applying, experiencing, and training closed hold. All seven breathing cycles are coordinated in four counts, breathing directly, fully, and calmly through the nose.

STARTING POSITION

Sit with your legs forward and your hands on your knees, with your back straight.

INITIAL INHALATION

Inhaling fully and calmly in four counts, extend your arms up and expand your chest well.

INITIAL EXHALATION

Exhaling fully and calmly in four counts, lie down on your back with your arms at your sides.

Synchronize the movement with your breathing, gradually rolling down the spine and coming to lie gently yet firmly on the floor at the end of the exhalation.

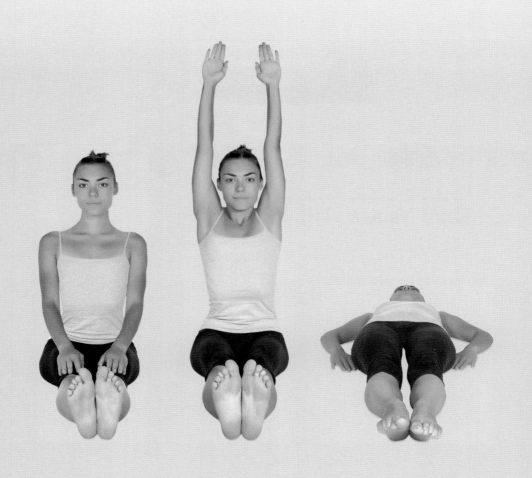

CENTRAL INHALATION

Inhaling fully and calmly in four counts, open your elbows slightly to the sides, leaving your palms on the floor, then raise your legs and torso up without bending your legs and bring your hands to your back to help you hold the position and straighten your torso well.

CLOSED HOLD

Holding closed for four counts, lower your knees and open them wide to join the soles of your feet together with your toes pointing upward. At the same time, move your hands to your knees and open them as far as possible while keeping your back straight, then stay in this position, which is reminiscent of a trident, supporting the weight of your body on your shoulders and the back of your head.

You may have to keep supporting your back with your hands rather than placing them on your knees to facilitate the correct alignment of your spine during the closed hold.

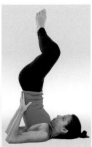

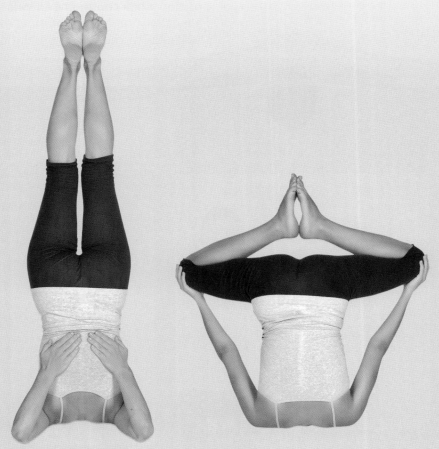

CENTRAL EXHALATION

At the end of the hold, roll forward and down, opening your legs wide as you exhale fully and calmly in four counts. Bend forward to bring your hands to your shins and your forehead to the floor.

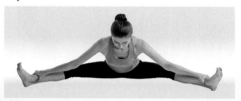

If you cannot bring your forehead to the floor, simply bend as far as possible without forcing, keeping your back straight.

CONCLUDING INHALATION

Inhaling fully and calmly in four counts, bring your legs together and extend your arms up, straightening your back and expanding your chest.

CONCLUDING EXHALATION

Exhaling fully and calmly in four counts, bring your forehead to your knees, lengthening your back from the root of your spine, and grasp the outsides of your feet.

REPETITION

To enjoy the full potential of the benefits of this Yantra, repeat the entire sequence two more times, either returning to the starting position while continuing to inhale and exhale calmly, or linking the final exhalation directly to the initial inhalation of the next round.

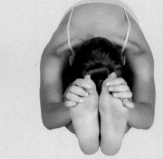

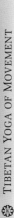

TRANSITION

To link the Trident to the next Yantra in the fourth series, the Tiger, inhale, rising back up from the concluding exhalation and stretching your arms over your head. Then exhale and place your hands on your knees.

HEALTH BENEFITS

- *Harmonizes the function of the five elements of the physical body*
- *Balances the force of the five pranas*
- *Restores digestive heat, a function of the fire-accompanying prana*
- *Counteracts problems caused by the damaged or disordered functioning of the ascending prana*

Related Warm-Ups (see Appendix 1): Butterfly (8), Soles Together Forward Bend (14), Open Forward Stretch (20), Spine Roll (30)

BREATHING CYCLE	COUNTS
Initial Inhalation	4
Initial Exhalation	4
Central Inhalation	4
Closed Hold	**4**
Central Exhalation	4
Concluding Inhalation	4
Concluding Exhalation	4

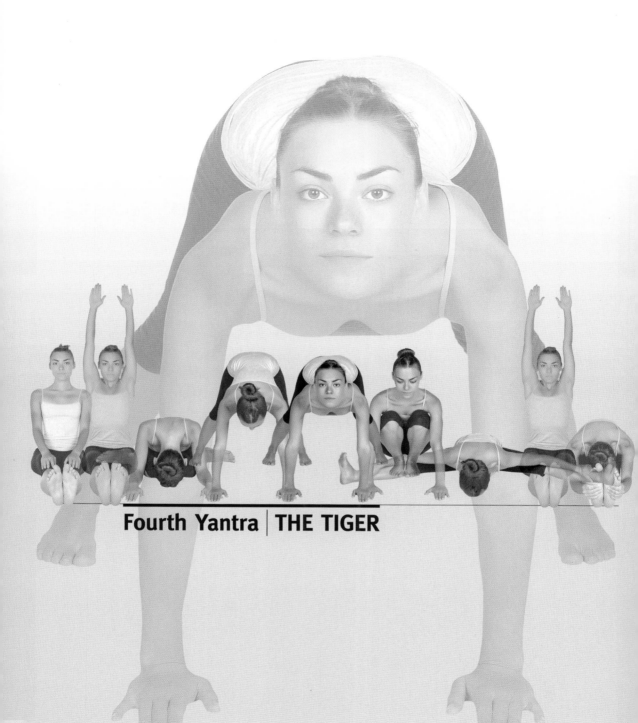

Fourth Yantra | THE TIGER

THE TIGER IS for the experience and training of contracted hold. The central inhalation is done in two counts, followed by a six-count contracted hold. All other cycles are performed to a count of four, breathing directly, fully, and calmly through the nose.

STARTING POSITION

Sit with your legs forward, hands on your knees, and your back straight.

Placing a thin cushion or firm prop beneath your buttocks may make the position and subsequent movements easier and more precise.

INITIAL INHALATION

Inhaling fully and calmly in four counts, stretch your arms over your head and open your chest well.

INITIAL EXHALATION

Exhaling fully and calmly in four counts, keep your knees joined while bringing your feet to the sides of your hips with your toes pointing to the sides. Then place your elbows next to the outside of your knees with your forearms and palms facing forward on the floor and parallel. Keep your spine straight and bring your forehead in front to the floor.

If you find it difficult to come into the position, you can bring your heels toward your perineum and roll forward onto your knees, as in the Turtle, separating your lower legs a little to sit between them with your buttocks on the floor and your toes ideally 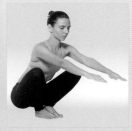 *pointing to the side. Then place your elbows next to the outside of your knees with your palms, forearms, and forehead to the floor.*

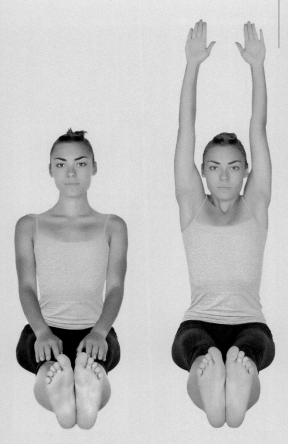

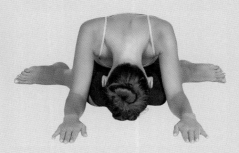

This position can be quite heavy on the knees. One way to make it softer is to leave your feet pointing backward along your thighs, but remember to open them outward 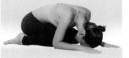 *a little when doing the next movement so that you can come into the correct position. If you still do not feel comfortable with the Tiger, do not do it. You can do the Dog instead for contracted hold. Another alternative is to start as in the* *second round of the Turtle, perhaps also using some props to be more comfortable and safe.*

CENTRAL INHALATION

Quickly inhaling directly in two counts, raise your torso up, keeping the soles of your feet and the palms of your hands firmly pressed on the floor.

CONTRACTED HOLD

Applying contracted hold for six counts, arch your head back and firmly push your abdomen against your spine as you straighten your back and remain in this pose, reminiscent of a tiger.

The dynamics of the movement make the experience of contracted hold particularly pronounced. The original Tibetan text uses the metaphor of pushing the "ocean" (the abdomen) against the "mountain" (the spine).

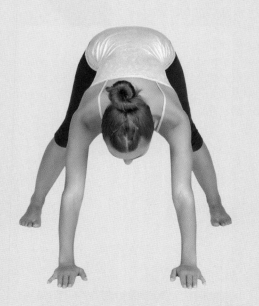

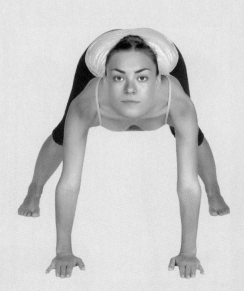

CENTRAL EXHALATION

Exhaling fully and calmly in four counts, bring your feet together with a soft jump and sit back on the floor, stretching your legs open and bringing your forearms along your legs and your hands to your shins while bending forward to bring your forehead toward or to the floor.

CONCLUDING INHALATION

Inhaling fully and calmly in four counts, bring your legs together in front of you and raise your arms over your head, opening your chest well.

CONCLUDING EXHALATION

Exhaling fully and calmly in four counts, bring your forehead to or toward your knees, lengthening your back from the root of your spine while firmly grasping the outsides of your feet with your hands.

REPETITION

To enjoy the full potential of the benefits of this Yantra, repeat the entire sequence two more times, either returning to the starting position while continuing to inhale and exhale calmly, or linking the final exhalation directly to the initial inhalation of the next round.

TRANSITION

To link the Tiger to the next Yantra in the fourth series, the Jewel, inhale, bringing your arms parallel above your head and keeping your back straight and your chest open. Exhale, bringing the soles of your feet together and placing your hands on your knees.

HEALTH BENEFITS

- *Alleviates ailments of the spine and spinal cord*
- *Improves the condition of the major and minor joints*
- *Relieves disorders of the nerves and ligaments of the head and limbs*
- *Eases sciatic pain*
- *Reduces stiffness*
- *Relieves conditions related to the small and large intestines and stomach*
- *Counteracts problems stemming from the deterioration of digestive heat due to imbalances of the fire-accompanying prana*

Related Warm-Ups (see Appendix 1): Rotating the Lower Legs (7), Hip and Knee Relaxer (11), Turning and Stretching (15), Knee Bend (16), Open Forward Stretch (20), Hip Releaser (26), Dog Training (36)

BREATHING CYCLE	COUNTS
Initial Inhalation	4
Initial Exhalation	4
Central Inhalation	2
Contracted Hold	**6**
Central Exhalation	4
Concluding Inhalation	4
Concluding Exhalation	4

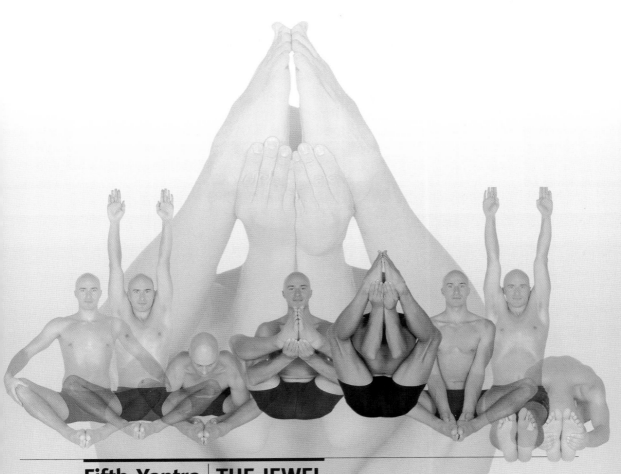

Fifth Yantra | THE JEWEL

THE JEWEL IS for experiencing and training empty hold. The central exhalation is done to two counts, followed by an empty hold for six counts. All other cycles are performed to four counts, breathing directly, fully, and calmly through the nose.

STARTING POSITION

Sit with the soles of your feet together and your hands on your knees. Your arms and back are straight and you are relaxed, present, and alert.

INITIAL INHALATION

Inhaling fully and calmly in four counts, stretch your arms up, expanding your chest well and keeping your back straight.

INITIAL EXHALATION

Exhaling fully and calmly in four counts, bend forward to bring your elbows under your knees and grasp your joined heels with the thumbs on top.

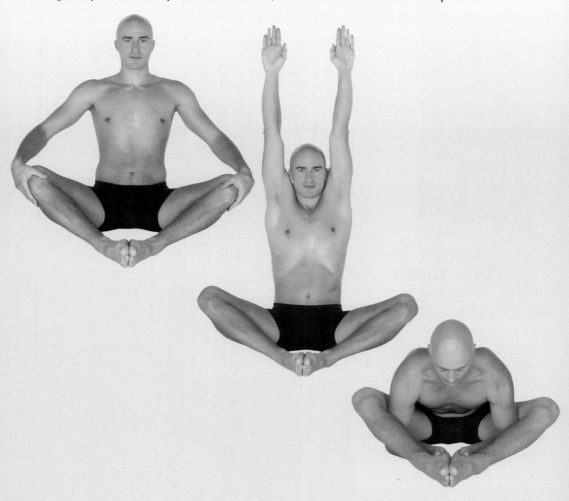

CENTRAL INHALATION

Inhaling fully and calmly in four counts, open your chest as you raise your joined feet to chest height, balancing on your buttocks.

CENTRAL EXHALATION

Exhaling with force in two counts, slowly push your feet toward the top of your head.

EMPTY HOLD

Remaining empty for six counts, tense your whole body and continue to straighten your back in this position, which is reminiscent of a jewel. Toward the end of the count, still holding empty, lower your hands and feet to the floor without separating them.

If balancing on your buttocks proves to be difficult, you can train near a wall or leaning on it to help support your back.

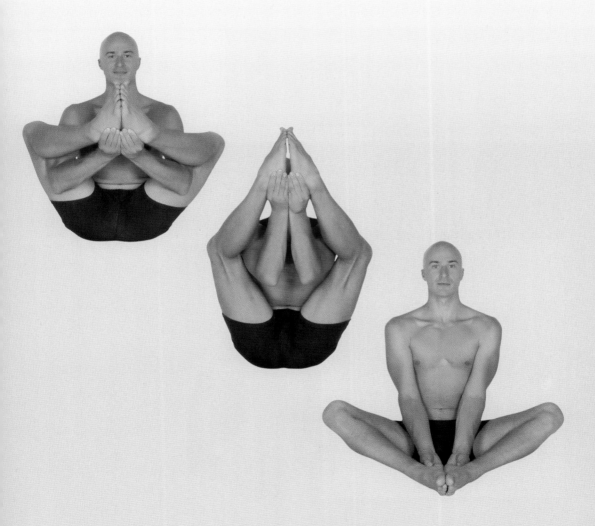

CONCLUDING INHALATION

Inhaling fully and calmly in four counts, extend your legs forward and parallel while raising your arms straight up, expanding your chest well.

CONCLUDING EXHALATION

Exhaling fully and calmly in four counts, bring your forehead to or toward your knees, lengthening your back from the root of your spine, and firmly grasp the outsides of your feet with your hands.

REPETITION

To enjoy the full potential of the benefits of this Yantra, repeat the entire sequence two more times, either returning to the starting position while continuing to inhale and exhale calmly, or linking the final exhalation directly to the initial inhalation of the next round.

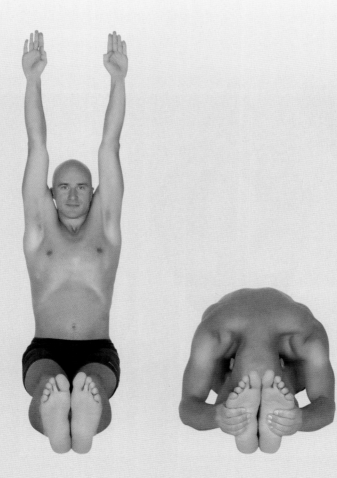

TRANSITION

If you are doing the fourth and fifth series in a single session, you can link the Jewel to the first Yantra of the fifth series, the Wheel, by inhaling as you raise your arms up over your head, then exhale and place your hands on your knees.

HEALTH BENEFITS

- *Harmonizes the condition of the five elements and the five pranas*
- *Alleviates problems caused by imbalances of the air, phlegm, and bile energies*
- *Increases physical strength*

Related Warm-Ups (see Appendix 1): Rotating the Legs (6), Rotating the Lower Legs (7), Both Knees to the Side Forward Bend (13), Soles Together Forward Bend (14)

BREATHING CYCLE	COUNTS
Initial Inhalation	4
Initial Exhalation	4
Central Inhalation	4
Central Exhalation	2
Empty Hold	**6**
Concluding Inhalation	4
Concluding Exhalation	4

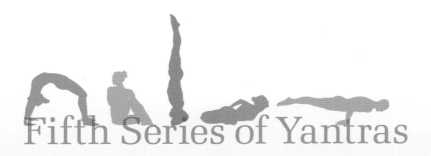

Fifth Series of Yantras

THE FIVE YANTRAS in the fifth series are the Wheel for open hold, the Eagle for directed hold, the Sword for closed hold, the Frog for contracted hold, and the Peacock for empty hold. The central phase of each Yantra in the fifth series features a quick two-count inhalation or exhalation followed by a six-count hold, while all other breathing cycles are done in four counts, breathing directly and calmly. If you find it difficult to practice in this rhythm, particularly the fast inhalation in two counts, you can do all seven cycles in four counts. As in the Yantras that end with a forward bending exhalation in the fourth series, we grab the sides of the feet instead of joining the fingers with the toes. The fifth series as a whole helps train and deepen the function of empty hold in particular.

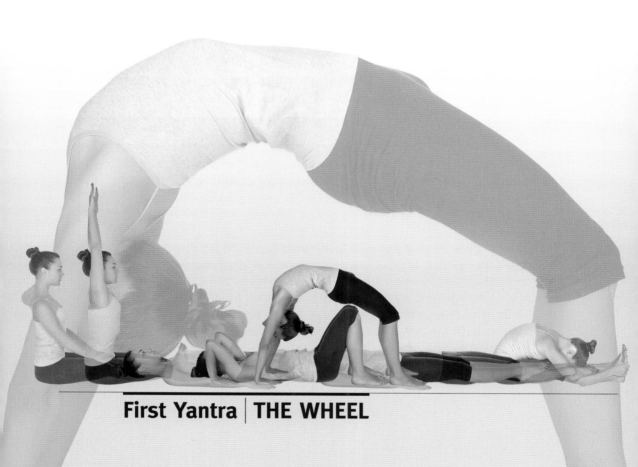

First Yantra | **THE WHEEL**

THE WHEEL IS for experiencing and training open hold. As in all of the Yantras for open hold, the chest and throat are stretched open so as not to block the retained air.

STARTING POSITION
Sit with your legs forward, your back straight, your hands on your knees, and your arms straight. You are present and relaxed.

INITIAL INHALATION
Inhaling calmly and fully in four counts, extend your arms up over your head.

INITIAL EXHALATION
Exhaling calmly and fully in four counts, lower your back gradually to the floor with intent and gentle control, bringing your arms along your sides with your palms on the floor.

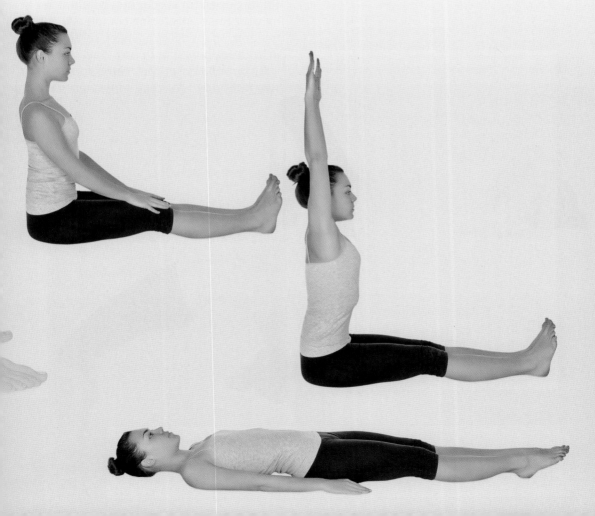

CENTRAL INHALATION

Inhaling in two counts, rotate your arms toward your head, placing your palms backward on the floor at shoulder level with your fingers pointing at your shoulders. At the same time, bend your legs to place your heels close to your buttocks. Still within the two-count inhalation, lift your pelvis and press your hands against the floor, straightening your elbows and coming up into a backward arch with your weight supported on your hands and feet. Your feet should stay parallel.

Do not force yourself to come into this position quickly if it does not feel comfortable and safe to you. As an alternative, you can extend the inhalation to four counts and shorten the subsequent open hold to four counts instead of six. You can also just arch enough to put the crown of your head on the floor and stay in open hold in that position. In both cases, most of your weight should be supported by your hands and feet.

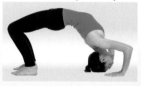

OPEN HOLD

Holding open for six counts, continue arching your torso, stretching completely in this position, shaped like a wheel, retaining the air without blocking in any way.

If you inhaled in four counts instead of two, hold open for only four counts.

CENTRAL EXHALATION

Exhaling calmly and fully in four counts, bend your elbows and your knees and turn your chin in the direction of your chest while you lower first your shoulders and then gradually your spine to the floor. As soon as your lower back reaches the floor, stretch your legs forward and bring your arms along your sides.

CONCLUDING INHALATION

Inhaling calmly and fully in four counts, bring your arms back and over your head, stretching from your fingers to your toes and tensing your whole body.

CONCLUDING EXHALATION

Exhaling calmly and fully in four counts, raise your torso up and forward as you bring your forehead to your knees and your hands to grasp the outsides of your feet.

REPETITION

To enjoy the full potential of the benefits of this Yantra, repeat the entire sequence two more times, either returning to the starting position while continuing to inhale and exhale calmly, or linking the final exhalation directly to the initial inhalation of the next round.

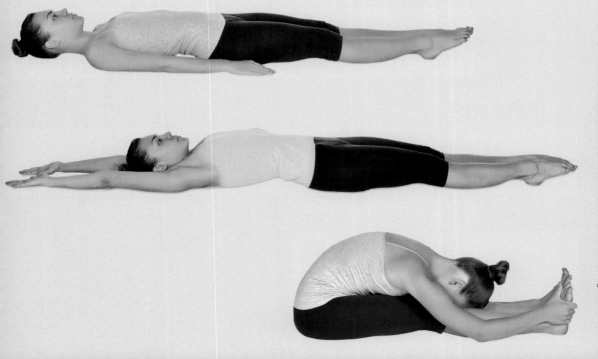

TRANSITION

To link the Wheel to the next Yantra in the fifth series, the Eagle, inhale, rising back up from the concluding exhalation and stretching your arms over your head. Then exhale and place your hands on your knees.

HEALTH BENEFITS

- *Alleviates imbalances of wind energy affecting the back, including problems with the spinal cord, the major and minor joints of the spine, and the muscles and tendons of the head and limbs*
- *Relieves lumbar pain, sciatic pain, and stiffness*
- *Restores the correct functioning of the pervasive prana when its functioning is disordered or impaired*

Related Warm-Ups (see Appendix 1): Bridge (29), Cat (31), Locust Training (32), Snake Training II (34), Neck Roll (37)

BREATHING CYCLE	COUNTS
Initial Inhalation	4
Initial Exhalation	4
Central Inhalation	2
Open Hold	**6**
Central Exhalation	4
Concluding Inhalation	4
Concluding Exhalation	4

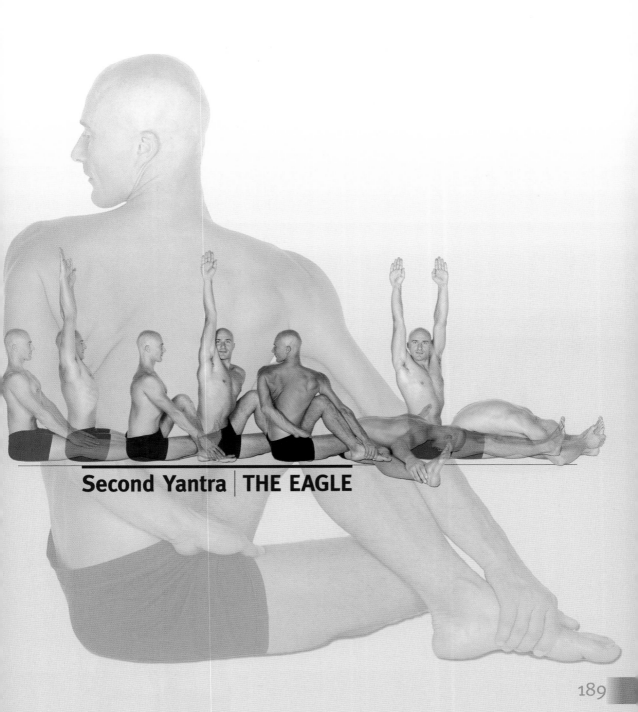

Second Yantra | THE EAGLE

THE EAGLE IS for experiencing and training directed hold. As in the first and second series, this Yantra accomplishes the directed hold through a spinal twist in its central phase. As an asymmetrical Yantra, women and men start on opposite sides.

STARTING POSITION

Sit with your legs forward, your hands on your knees, and your back straight.

INITIAL INHALATION

Inhaling calmly and fully in four counts, extend your arms straight over your head, expanding your chest well.

INITIAL EXHALATION

Exhaling calmly and fully in four counts, and using your hands to guide your feet into position, bend one leg and bring the heel to the opposite buttock while crossing your other leg over the thigh and bringing the other foot alongside the knee that is on the floor.

In the first round, women bend the left leg, bring the left heel to the right buttock, and cross the right foot over the left thigh, placing the right foot next to the left knee. Men bend the right leg, bring the right heel to the left buttock, and cross the left foot over the right thigh, placing the left foot next to the right knee.

CENTRAL INHALATION

Inhaling completely from the bottom up in two counts, raise your arm on the open side, energetically stretching the arm and your torso upward and opening your shoulders to expand your chest as you twist to the open side with your head straight.

In the first round, women raise the left arm and twist to the open side on the left. Men raise the right arm and twist to the open side on the right.

Like the inhalation, start the twisting movement from below and extend and expand with the torsion. Let the movement be guided by the twisting of your spine rather than the active movement of your shoulders. Do not push or force the twist.

DIRECTED HOLD

Direct the hold for six counts by keeping your spine aligned as you thoroughly twist your torso and head to the closed side while lowering your hand to grab the inside edge of your foot next to your knee. Wrap your other arm around your back, firmly grabbing onto your hip, and remain in this pose, like a majestically seated eagle.

In the first round, women twist to the right during the hold and men twist to the left.

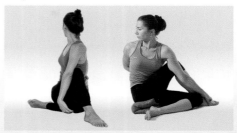

If you find this difficult to perform, a number of modifications are possible. The most important point is to keep your back and your sides straight and your lower back stable. Instead of grabbing the inside edge of your foot next to your knee, you can simply grab your ankle. Instead of wrapping your arm around your back, you can keep it straight out to the side to help you achieve the correct alignment of your back and the correct function of the hold. Additionally, placing a thin firm cushion beneath your buttocks can facilitate the positions and movements of this Yantra.

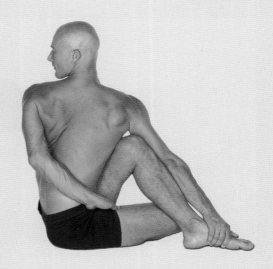

CENTRAL EXHALATION

Exhaling calmly and fully in four counts, extend your legs forward and apart, then place your forearms on your extended legs as you lower your forehead to or toward the floor.

CONCLUDING INHALATION

Inhaling calmly and fully in four counts, bring your legs together, raise your arms above your head, and expand your chest while gradually twisting and stretching your torso to the opposite side.

In the first round, women twist to the left and men twist to the right.

CONCLUDING EXHALATION

Exhaling calmly and fully in four counts, bend forward to bring your forehead to or toward your knees while firmly grabbing the outside edge of your feet.

REPETITION

Repeat the entire sequence on the opposite side, either returning to the starting position while continuing to inhale and exhale calmly, or linking the final exhalation directly to the initial inhalation of the second round. Then continue as before, but reversing the position of your arms and legs.

In the second round, women bring the right heel to the left buttock and the left foot next to the right knee. Men bring the left heel to the right buttock and the right foot next to the left knee.

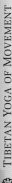

TRANSITION

To link the Eagle to the next Yantra in the fifth series, the Sword, inhale and raise your arms over your head. While exhaling, bring your heels toward your perineum while lowering your arms and rolling forward onto your knees to sit on your heels with the tops of your feet flat on the floor and your hands resting on your knees.

You can also cross your legs to roll forward into the kneeling position.

HEALTH BENEFITS

- *Alleviates ailments of the lumbar region and kidneys*
- *Improves the condition of the major and minor joints and the spine and spinal cord*
- *Relieves disorders of the head, arms, and legs*
- *Counteracts problems related to the sense organs*
- *Balances the five elements and five pranas*
- *Increases physical strength*
- *Enhances our capacity of body, voice, and mind*

Related Warm-Ups (see Appendix 1): Swinging (1), Knees to the Chest (9), Knees to the Side (10), Knee to the Side Forward Bend (12), Turning and Stretching (15), Crossed Knee Stretch (17), Knee over Knee (18), Leg Sweep (25), Supine Twist (27)

BREATHING CYCLE	COUNTS
Initial Inhalation	4
Initial Exhalation	4
Central Inhalation	2
Directed Hold	**6**
Central Exhalation	4
Concluding Inhalation	4
Concluding Exhalation	4

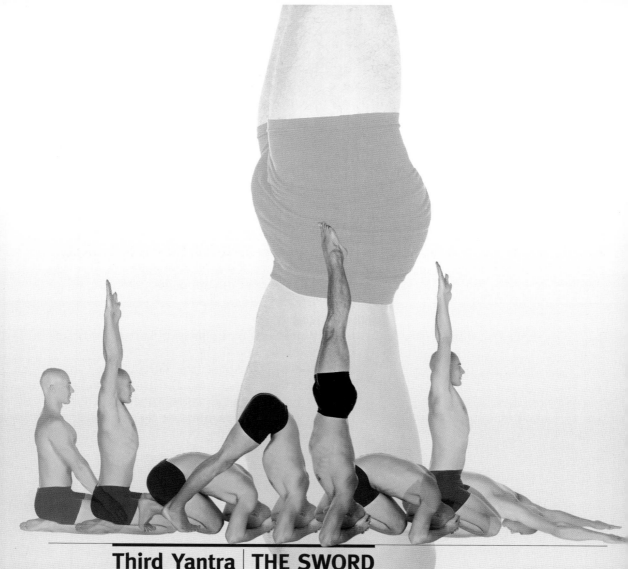

Third Yantra | **THE SWORD**

THE SWORD IS for experiencing and training closed hold. Once again, we have a two-count central inhalation followed by a six-count hold (in this case a closed hold), but if this is too difficult, both can be done in four counts. All other cycles are done in four counts, breathing fully and calmly.

Before performing this Yantra, it is important to practice the central inhalation movements until you feel comfortable coming up into the headstand. It can be helpful to train near a wall or with someone assisting you.

STARTING POSITION
Relaxed and present, sit on your heels with your hands on your knees and your back straight.

INITIAL INHALATION
Inhaling calmly and fully in four counts, extend your arms above your head, expanding your chest.

INITIAL EXHALATION
Exhaling calmly and fully in four counts, curl your toes under, lower your elbows and forearms to the floor, interlace your fingers, and place the upper part of your forehead on the floor at the apex of a triangle formed by your interlaced fingers and your open elbows.

One way to measure the proper distance between your elbows is to grab each elbow with the opposite hand, then maintain that distance as you open your arms and interlace your fingers.

CENTRAL INHALATION

Inhaling in two counts, straighten your knees and extend your legs as you raise them straight up, evenly distributing your weight on your forearms, elbows, and forehead at the hairline, the harder part of the skull.

You may find it helpful to take four counts to come up, and then hold for four counts instead of six. If necessary, you can bend your knees first and then straighten your legs, in this case not inhaling to your full capacity but favoring the 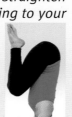 *abdominal phase of the breathing over the chest phase. Do not practice this Yantra lightly if you have a problem with blood pressure, your neck, or any other medical condition that would make it inadvisable.*

As mentioned above, it is crucial to practice this phase until you are comfortable coming up into headstand (see end of chapter for training instructions).

CLOSED HOLD

Holding closed for six counts, keep stretching your legs and feet upward with the inside edges of your feet joined, remaining in this position, which resembles the shape of the sword of wisdom.

As mentioned earlier, you can also hold for only four counts if you are not comfortable with holding for six counts. It is important never to force or strain your body or your breathing. Practice with intent and let the movements flow with relaxed and harmonious energy.

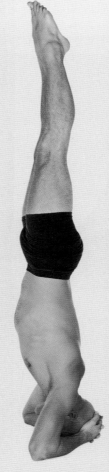

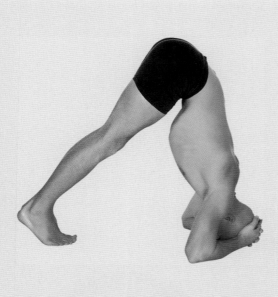

CENTRAL EXHALATION
Exhaling calmly and fully in four counts, slowly lower your extended legs, bringing your knees to the floor and curling your toes under.

CONCLUDING INHALATION
Inhaling calmly and fully in four counts, raise your torso upright and extend your arms above your head.

CONCLUDING EXHALATION
Exhaling calmly and fully in four counts, remain seated on your heels as you bring the tops of your feet flat on the floor, stretch your arms in front of your knees, and bring your forehead to the floor.

REPETITION
To enjoy the full potential of the benefits of this Yantra, repeat the entire sequence two more times, either returning to the starting position while continuing to inhale and exhale calmly, or linking the final exhalation directly to the initial inhalation of the next round.

TRANSITION

To link the Sword to the next Yantra in the third series, the Frog, inhale, rising back up and stretching your arms over your head. Then exhale and place your hands on your knees.

TRAINING FOR THE SWORD

A good way to train, near a wall if you like, is to take the position described in the initial exhalation, then raise your buttocks up, keeping your knees bent and feet on the floor, and walk toward your chest until you find the balance to allow you to lift your thighs against your chest. At this point you can stretch your legs up in a gradual, straight, and controlled manner.

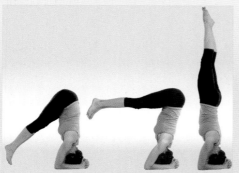

Once you are comfortable coming up this way, you can try walking toward your chest while keeping your legs straight and, when you find the right balance, lift your legs up without bending them. Do not try to jump up by throwing your legs in the air; it can be dangerous for your neck and spine.

- *Sharpens the intellectual faculties*
- *Promotes mental lucidity*
- *Alleviates problems related to the impaired functioning of the nerves of the five sense organs and the brain*
- *Restores balance to the five pranas and five elements*
- *Reinforces and fosters the correct functioning of the wind, bile, and phlegm energies*

Breathing Cycle	Counts
Initial Inhalation	4
Initial Exhalation	4
Central Inhalation	2
Closed Hold	**6**
Central Exhalation	4
Concluding Inhalation	4
Concluding Exhalation	4

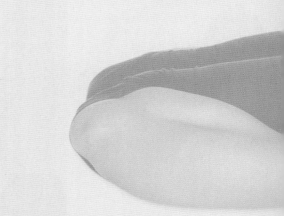

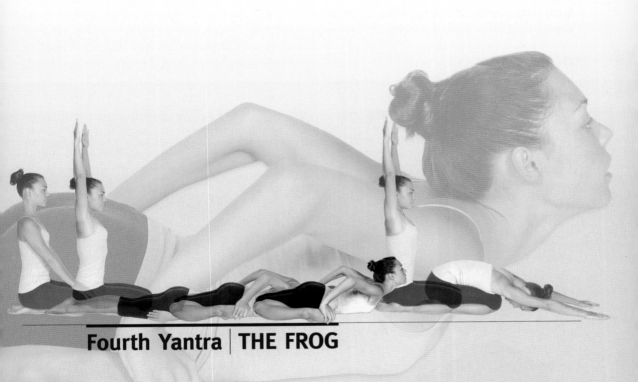

Fourth Yantra | **THE FROG**

THE FROG IS for experiencing and training contracted hold, in this case an empty contracted hold. In this Yantra, we exhale before the hold for two counts and then apply directed hold for six counts as we contract the abdomen toward the spine. If the two- and six-count timing is too difficult, the exhalation and hold can both be done in four counts. All other cycles are done in four counts, breathing fully and calmly.

STARTING POSITION
Sit on your heels with your hands on your knees and your back straight.

INITIAL INHALATION
Inhaling calmly and fully in four counts, stretch your arms up over your head, expanding and opening your chest.

INITIAL EXHALATION
Exhaling calmly and fully in four counts, stretch your arms straight forward and place your palms on the floor in front of you, then come into a prone position with your arms along your sides and your forehead on the floor.

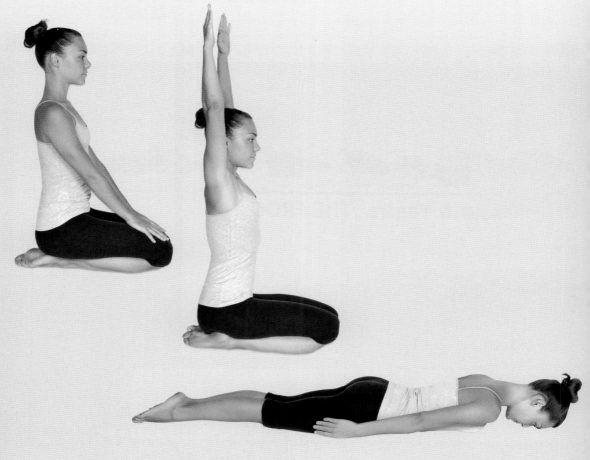

CENTRAL INHALATION

Inhaling calmly and fully in four counts, raise your arms up and back as you bend your legs toward your buttocks, then grasp the outsides of your feet and rotate your hands, joining the thumbs and your big toes, with your palms on your forefoot and your fingers around the toes.

CENTRAL EXHALATION

In two counts, while quickly emitting an aspirated "HA" sound, contract your buttocks, arch your head and torso up and back, and open your elbows while pressing your feet to the floor by your sides.

If you cannot bring your feet to the floor, press only as far as is comfortable. Do not force yourself to go beyond your capacity in any way. You can also just grab your feet from the inside and lower them as much as you can while keeping your elbows open.

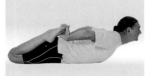

CONTRACTED HOLD

Applying an empty contracted hold for six counts, remain in this position, reminiscent of a frog, as you draw your sides and your abdomen in toward your spine.

In this Yantra, the contracted hold is empty.

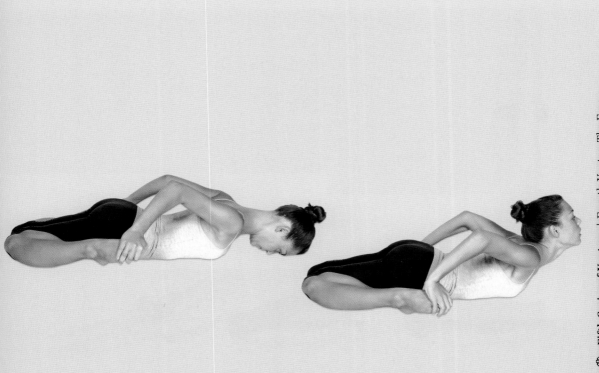

CONCLUDING INHALATION

Inhaling calmly and fully in four counts, place your hands at the sides of your chest as you stretch your legs out, roll back, sit on your heels with the tops of your feet on the floor, and stretch your arms up, expanding your chest well.

CONCLUDING EXHALATION

Exhaling calmly and fully in four counts, stretch your arms forward as you bend to bring your forehead and your arms to the floor in front of you.

REPETITION

To enjoy the full potential of the benefits of this Yantra, repeat the entire sequence two more times, either returning to the starting position while continuing to inhale and exhale calmly, or linking the final exhalation directly to the initial inhalation of the next round.

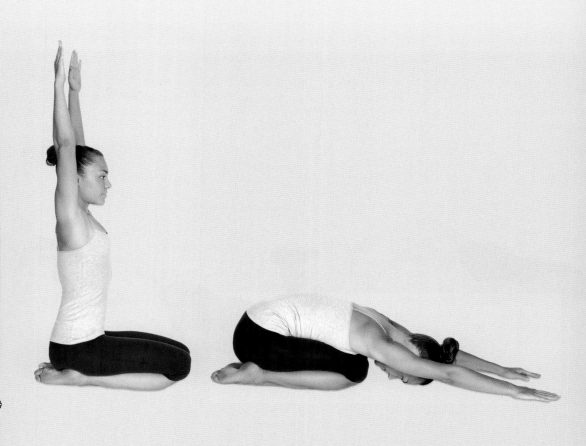

TRANSITION

To link the Frog to the next Yantra in the third series, the Peacock, inhale, rising back up to sit with your back straight and your arms over your head. Then exhale and place your hands on your knees.

HEALTH BENEFITS

- *Balances and harmonizes the functions of the five elements*
- *Strengthens the solid and hollow organs*
- *Alleviates problems related to malfunctioning of the solid and hollow organs*
- *Relieves disorders related to the fire-accompanying and downward-clearing pranas*
- *Aids the processes of digestion and elimination*

Related Warm-Ups (see Appendix 1): Swinging (1), Crossed Knee Stretch (17), Knee over Knee (18), Supine Twist (27)

BREATHING CYCLE	COUNTS
Initial Inhalation	4
Initial Exhalation	4
Central Inhalation	4
Central Exhalation	2
Contracted Empty Hold	**6**
Concluding Inhalation	4
Concluding Exhalation	4

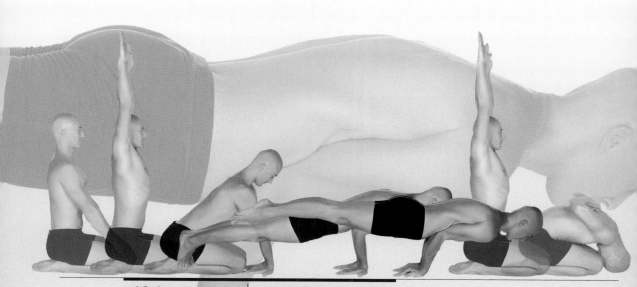

Fifth Yantra | THE PEACOCK

T HE PEACOCK IS for experiencing and training empty hold. The exhalation before the hold is for two counts and the empty hold is for six. As with the other Yantras in the fifth series, if the combination of the short exhalation and long hold is too difficult, both can be done in four counts instead. All other cycles are done in four counts, breathing fully and calmly.

STARTING POSITION

Sit on your heels with your hands on your knees, your back straight, and your shoulders relaxed and open.

INITIAL INHALATION

Inhaling calmly and fully in four counts, extend your arms up over your head, expanding your chest well.

INITIAL EXHALATION

Exhaling calmly and fully in four counts, place your palms backward on the floor with your fingertips just in front of your knees.

If it helps with the next movement, you can place your hands between your slightly open knees.

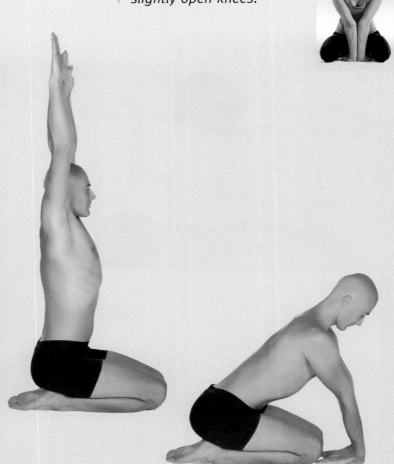

CENTRAL INHALATION

Inhaling calmly and fully in four counts, extend your legs behind you, open your chest, and balance your body on your hands and the tips of your toes as you join your elbows and press them firmly into your abdomen.

CENTRAL EXHALATION

Forcefully exhaling in two counts, slightly shift your balance forward, keeping your elbows well pressed into your abdomen. Then lift your extended legs off the floor, supporting the weight of your body with your hands and forearms.

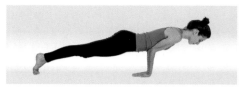

Keeping your torso and body straight as an arrow will help you accomplish the lift. If you find it too difficult to come off the floor, you can leave your toes on the floor while keeping your body well controlled and straight.

EMPTY HOLD

Holding empty for six counts, remain suspended on your hands and forearms in this pose, reminiscent of a peacock, keeping your legs extended and straight.

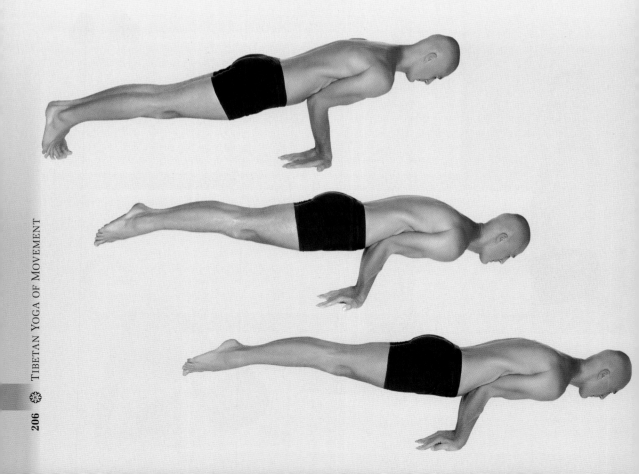

CONCLUDING INHALATION

Inhaling calmly and fully in four counts, bring your knees to the floor and sit back on your heels as you stretch your arms over your head, expanding your chest.

CONCLUDING EXHALATION

Exhaling calmly and fully in four counts, join the palms of your hands behind your back and bend forward, bringing your forehead to your knees.

REPETITION

To enjoy the full potential of the benefits of this Yantra, repeat the entire sequence two more times, either returning to the starting position while continuing to inhale and exhale calmly, or linking the final exhalation directly to the initial inhalation of the next round.

HEALTH BENEFITS

- *Strengthens the main nerves of the five solid organs and six hollow organs*
- *Enhances the functioning of the five elements of the physical body*
- *Restores balance to the five pranas when their functions are disordered or damaged*

Related Warm-Up (see Appendix 1): Arm Stretch (41)

BREATHING CYCLE	COUNTS
Initial Inhalation	4
Initial Exhalation	4
Central Inhalation	4
Central Exhalation	2
Empty Hold	**6**
Concluding Inhalation	4
Concluding Exhalation	4

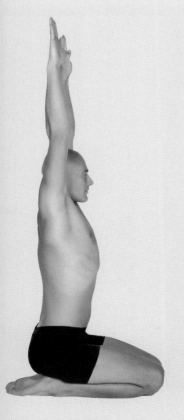

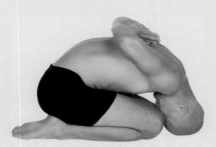

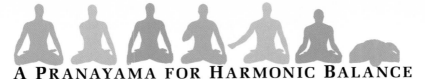

A PRANAYAMA FOR HARMONIC BALANCE

Rhythmic Breathing

RHYTHMIC BREATHING IS a pranayama that effectively trains us to coordinate and improve the individual phases of the process of breathing. The balanced ratio between inhalation, open hold, and exhalation, followed by an empty hold, helps expand our breathing capacity while making our respiration calmer and more complete, allowing us to train to breathe in a conscious, continuous, uninterrupted, and natural flow. Because the rhythm of our heartbeat is connected with our respiration, Rhythmic Breathing is a particularly effective means to coordinate this function. Especially when we apply a rhythm where the exhalation is longer than the inhalation, the heartbeat slows down and we experience a relaxing effect. It balances our energy, calms stress and nervousness, and counteracts depression.

When practicing Rhythmic Breathing, it is important to maintain presence without distraction, mindfully following the flow of the breath while focusing your attention on the four phases of the breathing: inhalation, open hold, exhalation, and empty hold. In Rhythmic Breathing, we count the rhythm with our right hand (the same hand for both genders). For the basic count of four, we first touch the left knee, then the right knee, then the center of the chest, finally opening the arm out to the side and clicking our fingers above the right knee. It is a simple but effective method to count the rhythm, and it is easy to learn. You can also use a metronome, but the steady movement of the hand has the advantage of helping the mind remain calm and concentrated.

The rhythm starts at four counts, with each count ideally corresponding to, or at least not faster than, the heartbeat of a healthy person when relaxed. Start by training with an even 4–4–4 count, counting four beats on the inhalation, four beats for the open hold, and four beats (two plus two) for the exhalation and empty hold. Get acquainted with this basic rhythm, and then gradually progress to 4–6–4, 4–8–4, and so on, following the increments specified in the table below. There is no prescribed number of repetitions before progressing to the next increment, but do not increase the count until you are fully comfortable with the previous stage. If at any time you feel any difficulty or tension, or before increasing the count, it is best to "change the air" by bending over and exhaling deeply one to three times, as in the last three phases of the Nine Purification Breathings. When the rhythm calls for a count of 6, 10, 14, or 18, or in other words, a number that is not a multiple of four, you have to add two beats by again touching the center of your chest and then opening your hand out to the side over your right knee and clicking your fingers.

Until the count of 4–16–8, the inhalation and exhalation are always direct. But when the count for the inhalation moves to six beats and higher, we can incorporate the indirect breathing method introduced in the Tsadul pranayama. When we use indirect breathing, at the beginning of the inhalation we gently control how we draw the air in, slightly tightening the glottis so that the breathing becomes faintly sonorous, then opening the glottis toward the end of the cycle to let the breathing flow directly again. It may help to think of the inhalation as the shape of a grain of barley or rice: slender at the beginning, stronger in the middle, and gently tapering off at the end. The other phases of the breathing remain the same. The phase of the hold stays open and relaxed. The exhalation-hold phase is always half direct exhalation and half relaxed, empty hold.

As with any other aspect of Yantra Yoga, when doing Rhythmic Breathing it is important not to force but to develop your capacity with training. Be kind to yourself. Not forcing does not mean being passive; it means you respect yourself and give space to your physical energy and your mind so that you can relax and progress in a steady, harmonious, and joyful way.

If you find the phase of indirect breathing challenging, it is also possible to inhale smoothly in a direct and slow way like we normally breathe in all of the Yantras. If you prefer, you can apply this wonderful breathing practice using the same table of progressive increments to train only the phases of inhalation and exhalation, without any hold. Beyond learning to breathe in a deeper and calmer way, it is important to train the flexibility of our breathing so we can gain the capacity to breathe in different ways and lengths with the same command and ease.

STARTING POSITION

Sit in the position of Vairochana or one of the alternatives described in the chapter on the Nine Purification Breathings. The main thing is that you are comfortable, with your back straight, your shoulders open, and your hands on your knees. If you are doing this pranayama as a standalone practice, begin by thoroughly exhaling the stale air by means of the Nine Purification Breathings, or at least the last three cycles of that exercise.

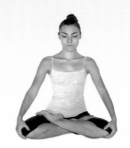

INHALATION CYCLE

Counting the respective beat for the inhalation cycle with your right hand, inhale completely, starting from your abdomen and expanding up into your chest, directly, smoothly, and calmly drawing in the air through your nose.

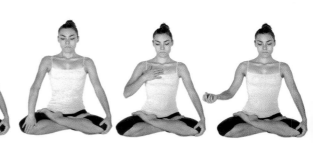

Count the beat by touching your right hand to your left knee, right knee, and the center of your chest, and then clicking your fingers above your right knee. In the beginning, start with a rhythm of 4–4–4. Refer to the table below for subsequent increments. For increments that include a beat or beats that are not multiples of four, repeat the last two motions of your hand for the correct count.

HOLD CYCLE

Counting the respective beat for the hold cycle with your right hand, retain the air in a relaxed and open hold, allowing it to expand freely.

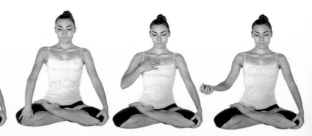

The hold should be like a relaxed pause in the flow of the breathing, without tension or any kind of blockage or obstruction. In Rhythmic Breathing, the hold phase is crucial. It is

profoundly effective in coordinating our energy and increasing our clarity of mind and our ability to focus.

EXHALATION CYCLE

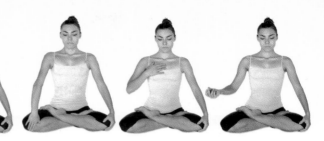

Counting the respective beat for the exhalation and empty hold cycle with your right hand, exhale for half of the cycle, initially increasing the flow of air, then decreasing it and entering into an empty hold for the second half of the cycle count.

When you are in empty hold, remain relaxed and calm, without blocking or tensing.

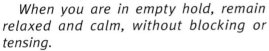

TABLE OF BREATHING CYCLES FOR RHYTHMIC BREATHING								
(I = Inhalation, OH = Open Hold, E+EH = Exhalation plus Empty Hold)								
I	OH	E + EH	I	OC	E + EH	I	OH	E + EH
4	4	4	6	14	10	8	14	12
4	6	4	6	16	10	8	16	12
4	8	4	6	18	10	8	18	12
4	6	6	6	20	10	8	20	12
4	8	6	6	12	12	8	22	12
4	10	6	6	14	12	8	24	12
4	12	6	6	16	12			
4	8	8	6	18	12			
4	10	8	6	20	12			
4	12	8	6	22	12			
4	14	8	6	24	12			
4	16	8						
			8	8	8			
6	6	6	8	10	8			
6	8	6	8	12	8			
6	10	6	8	14	8			
6	12	6	8	16	8			
6	8	8	8	10	10			
6	10	8	8	12	10			
6	12	8	8	14	10			
6	14	8	8	16	10			
6	16	8	8	18	10			
6	10	10	8	20	10			
6	12	10	8	12	12			

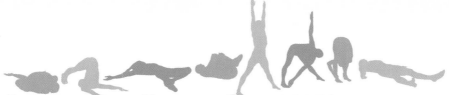

The Vajra Wave

THE VAJRA WAVE is a sequence of movements to be performed at the end of every session of Yantra Yoga. Synchronizing strong, direct inhalations and exhalations with each and every phase of movement, its purpose is to help us overcome any obstacles affecting our breathing and energy. It has the capacity to coordinate the functions of our elements and to balance excessively strong or weak prana and other imbalances of the pranic energy.

In all phases of the sequence, the breathing is strong and direct, uninterrupted, without any holds or microholds whatsoever. The movements are rhythmic and energetic, without a specific count but with a continuous, regular, symmetrical pace of breathing and movement. All movements are done with presence and energy, with intent. Women and men start the asymmetrical phases on opposite sides, without alternating in subsequent rounds.

As a quicker and easier alternative to the Vajra Wave, you can also end your session with three or seven exhalations: Starting from a standing position, simply stretch your arms straight up over your head with an energetic inhalation, then bend forward, swinging your arms down with an energetic exhalation. If you like, you can bend your legs a little when exhaling to make it softer on your lower back. Repeat for a total of seven cycles of inhalation and exhalation, and finally lie down to relax.

THE PRACTICE

1 Sit on the floor with your legs extended, hands on your knees, and your back straight.

2 Inhale strongly, directly, and quickly as you raise your arms up over your head.

3 Exhale, bringing the soles of your feet together near your perineum and bending your head and torso forward toward the floor as you stretch your arms back along your sides.

4 Inhale and lie on your back, straightening your legs in front of you and bringing your arms to the floor straight over your head.

5 Exhale, bringing your arms in front by your sides and swinging your legs straight over your head, as in the Plow Yantra.

If you find this phase difficult to perform or want to make it gentler on your lower back, instead of lying back in phase 4, inhale and stretch your legs out straight as you raise your arms over your head. Then exhale and help yourself roll down in phase 5, bringing your legs over your head and your arms along your sides, as in the Plow Yantra.

6 Inhale, bringing your legs forward and your arms out to the sides while opening all four limbs wide apart.

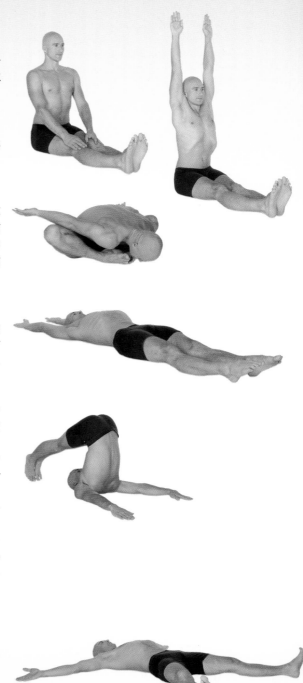

7 Exhale, keeping your torso and pelvis on the floor, and energetically strike the inside of your elbow with the opposite hand and the side of your knee with the sole of the opposite foot, keeping the knee of the active leg as low as possible.

In each round, women start by striking the inside of the right elbow with the left hand and the side of the right knee with the left foot. Men strike the inside of the left elbow with the right hand and the side of the left knee with the right foot.

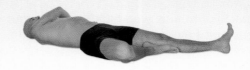

8 Inhale as you press your hand into your arm, strongly massage from the inside of your elbow across your chest, and open your arm out to the side, simultaneously pressing your foot into your leg and pulling it from the side of your knee to the top of your thigh, then opening the leg wide again.

It is also possible to make the massage stronger by using the vajra fists instead of open hands.

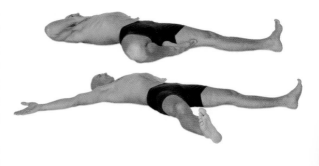

9 Exhale, energetically striking the inside of your other elbow with your other hand and the side of your other knee with the sole of your other foot.

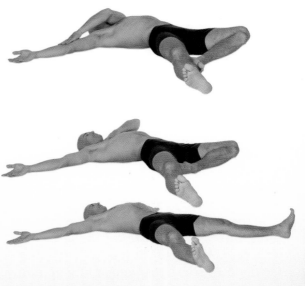

10 Inhale as you press your hand into your arm and strongly massage from the inside of your elbow up the arm and across your chest all the way to your side, simultaneously pressing your foot into your leg and pulling it from the side of your knee to the top of your thigh. Then open the leg wide again.

11 Exhale, bringing your hands around your knees and hugging them to your chest.

12 Inhale, rolling forward with your hands around your knees and coming into a standing position with your arms over your head, the soles of your feet on the floor, and your legs two cubits apart.

To make it easier and less stressful on your knees, you can come into the standing position with your feet together and then step two cubits to the side.

13 Exhale as you bend forward, twist your torso to one side, and bring the fingers of one hand to the opposite toes, keeping your other arm straight up and gazing at the fingertips of your elevated hand.

In each round, women twist to the left and bring the fingers of the right hand to the left foot. Men twist to the right and bring the fingers of the left hand to the right foot.

Keep your legs straight; do not bend them. Keeping your legs wide apart makes it easier to perform this position correctly.

14 Inhale, raising your torso up and extending both arms parallel over your head.

15 Exhale as you bend forward, twist your torso to the other side, and bring the fingers of the other hand to the opposite toes, keeping your other arm straight up and gazing at the fingertips of your elevated hand.

In this step, women twist to the right and bring the fingers of the left hand to the right foot. Men twist to the left and bring the fingers of the right hand to the left foot.

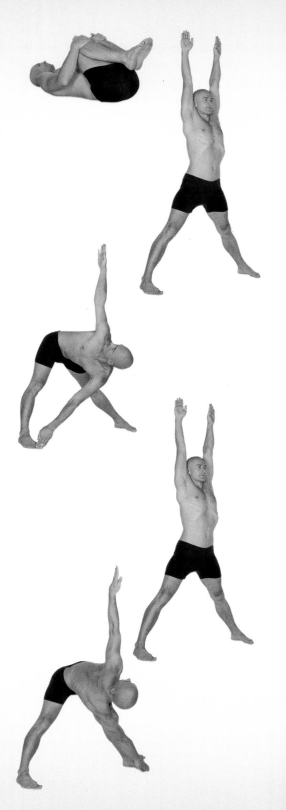

16 Inhale, straightening your torso, extending your arms over your head, and bringing your legs parallel.

Keep your feet slightly apart to have better balance.

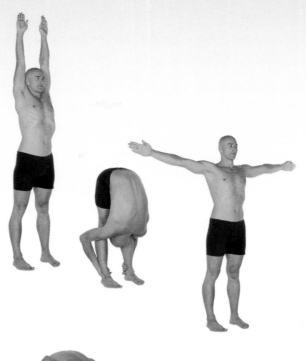

17 Exhale, bending forward, grabbing your ankles with your hands, and bringing your forehead to your knees.

If possible, keep your legs straight; if this is too difficult, you can bend them a little.

18 Inhale, raising your torso straight up and opening your arms wide apart to form a T.

19 Exhale and sit on your heels, joining the palms of your hands with the soles of your feet, and bending your torso forward.

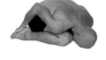

To keep the correct even pace throughout the exercise, it might be necessary to do this movement a bit faster than the other phases. In this phase, try to observe whether you have a tendency to hold your breath and exhale only at the end of the movement. When performed correctly, the breath is not held at any time in the Vajra Wave. By avoiding fragmenting the breathing with even small holds, you can perform the exercise in a strong, harmonious, and continuous flow of movement and breathing, allowing it to fulfill its purpose of eliminating obstacles affecting the pranic energy.

20 Inhale, rolling back to bring your buttocks to the floor as you join the soles of your feet in front of your perineum, ending the movement by stretching your arms up over your head.

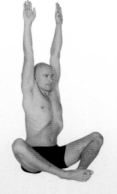

REPETITION

If possible, it is best to repeat the Vajra Wave three, five, or seven times, but even a single sequence is beneficial. When repeating it, continue from phase 20 to phase 3 without interrupting the flow of the movement. At the beginning of subsequent rounds, the soles of your feet will already be joined when you exhale and lean forward.

CONCLUSION

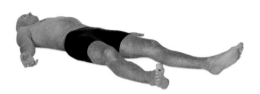

When you want to conclude your practice of the Vajra Wave, after stretching your arms up at the end of phase 20, exhale forcefully and lie down on your back with your legs and feet apart and your arms loosely out to the side, abandoning any tension in your body.

RELAXATION

Inhaling and exhaling naturally, relax completely, and continue to inhale and exhale slowly, deeply, and naturally, without modifying anything. Let all tensions in your body relax. Let your breathing be spontaneous and relaxed. Let your mind be free and relaxed. Let everything be in its authentic, natural, and harmonious condition.

When our energy is really coordinated, harmonized, and in tune with the body and mind, we can finally experience a state of true relaxation.

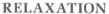

Appendix 1
A Selection of Pre-Practice Warm-Ups

BEFORE BEGINNING A session of Yantra Yoga, it can be useful to do some simple exercises to warm up the body. Warming up will facilitate a more correct and comfortable sitting position and help you perform the various sequences of movements with greater ease. Although these exercises are not part of Vairochana's original instructions on Yantra Yoga, they have become part of the general approach to the practice. They are especially useful if you are fairly new to yoga or are not able to practice as often as you would like. In addition to training the body for specific Yantras, warm-ups are a good way to shake off tension and stress.

The exercises selected here address six main actions to harmoniously warm up and train the overall flexibility and tone of the body, and especially the spine: bending forward, arching backward, stretching the left side, stretching the right side, twisting to the left, and twisting to the right. If you have decided to concentrate on a particular series of Yantras during your session of practice, you can focus on warm-up exercises that will make those movements easier to perform and more precise. We have listed corresponding Yantras and movement types for the individual warm-ups to help you identify the exercises most relevant for your practice.

You do not need to do all the warm-up exercises suggested here, and in fact it is best to keep the length of your warm-up session in proportion to the actual practice of Yantra Yoga. Taking into account the amount of time you have, choose the warm-ups that are most effective for you. Whenever possible, coordinate your breathing with the movements. Let your inhalations and exhalations be relaxed, but filled with a sense of presence and energy, full of life. In almost all of the warm-ups, the quality of the breathing is complete, calm, and smooth. In general, inhale when the movement is expanding and exhale when closing or contracting.

Standing Warm-Ups

Start with a few standing poses if you like.

1. SWINGING

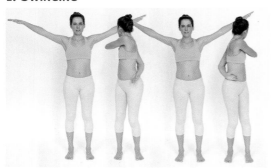

Stand relaxed yet present, feet parallel and at least a shoulder-width apart, and inhale, opening your arms wide to the side. Exhale and swing your arms around your hips, turning to one side and rotating your spine, letting your arms hang loose so that your hands alternately slap against the sides of your body as you swing. Inhale, coming back to the center while opening your arms wide to the side. Then exhale, turning to the other side. Repeat three to five times.

Training Focus: All movements involving torsion, in particular the 4th Tsigjong, the 3rd and 8th Lungsangs, the Conch, the Curved Knife, and the Eagle

2. TREE

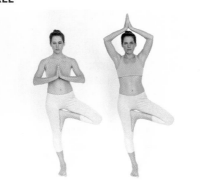

Stand relaxed yet present with your feet slightly apart and parallel, your arms along your sides. Use your hand to bring the sole of one foot to the top of the inner thigh of your other leg. Breathe calmly and balance on your standing leg. Focusing on an unmoving spot in the distance will help you maintain your balance. Join your palms in front of your chest and slowly raise your joined hands above your head, standing on one leg as long as the pose is comfortable and easy. Then slowly bring your joined hands back down to your chest as you lower your foot to the floor. Return to the starting position with your arms along your sides and then repeat on the other side, alternating several times.

Training Focus: All movements involving balancing in general, in particular the 2nd Tsadul

3. SQUAT

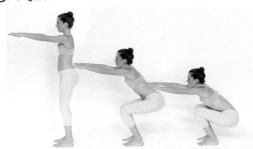

Stand relaxed yet present with your feet slightly apart and parallel, arms along your sides. Inhale, bringing your arms parallel in front at shoulder level. Exhale as you bend your knees and squat down toward your heels, going only as far as is comfortable and keeping your feet as flat on the floor as possible. Inhale, rising back up and keeping your arms in front. Repeat three to five times.

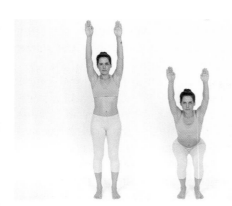

(a) Standing straight again, inhale, this time raising your arms straight up over your head, vertical from your shoulders and parallel. Squat down toward your heels as you exhale, keeping your back and your arms straight. Keep your arms stretched up, reaching vigorously and counterbalancing the downward stretch at the base of your spine. Inhale, rising back up. Exhale and slowly squat down toward your heels. Repeat three to five times.

Training Focus: All movements involving rising up and down, in particular the Dagger, the Half-Moon, and the Vulture

Seated Warm-Ups

When doing seated exercises, it is important to keep your back as straight as possible, without forcing or creating unwanted tension, but at the same time maintaining tone and energy.

4. SHAKING THE FEET
Sitting on the floor with your back straight and your legs parallel in front, grab one foot by the ankle with both hands, bring it in front of your torso, and shake it vigorously. Stretch the leg in front, then grab and shake the other foot. Continue to alternate for three to five repetitions.

Let your breathing be continuous and relaxed, inhaling and exhaling through your nose. Keep your feet loose and relaxed and your shoulders open.

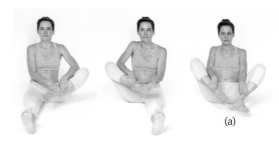

(a)

(a) Now grab both feet and shake them vigorously while balancing on your buttocks.

Training Focus: All movements actively involving the feet, in particular the 2nd Tsigjong

5. SWINGING THE LOWER LEGS

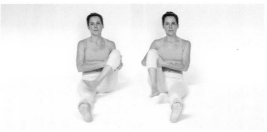

Sitting on the floor with both legs stretched in front or one leg bent so that your foot is near your perineum, grab your other leg above the knee joint with both hands, interlace your fingers, and swing your lower leg from side to side three to five times, keeping the leg and knee joint loose and relaxed. Repeat with the other leg, alternating several times.

Training Focus: All movements involving the knee joints and ankles

6. ROTATING THE LEGS

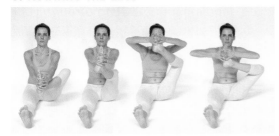

Sitting with your legs straight, grasp one foot firmly with both hands and inhale as you guide your foot up toward your forehead, then exhale as you lower it close to your body, down to the level of your navel. In this exercise, you basically draw large circles with your foot on a plane perpendicular to the center of your body. Repeat three to five times, then switch sides.

Training Focus: All movements involving knee and hip joints, in particular the 3rd Tsigjong, the Spider, and the Jewel

7. ROTATING THE LOWER LEGS

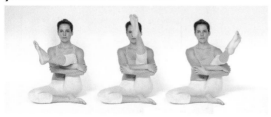

Sitting with one foot at your perineum, raise your other knee up and cradle it on your arms, clasping each arm just above the elbow or the wrists with your opposite hand. Keeping your back as straight as possible, inhale and exhale as you rotate your lower leg, drawing large circles in the air in front of you with your foot, first three to five times in one direction, then in the other. Then switch sides.

Training Focus: All movements involving knee joints and hamstrings, in particular the Tiger and the Jewel

8. BUTTERFLY

Sit with your back straight, your knees open, and the soles of your feet together with your heels close to your perineum. Keep your arms stretched along your sides, supporting yourself behind your back with your hands in fists or just flat on the floor. Keep your shoulders open and your back straight. Bounce your knees up and down toward the floor, opening as much as possible. Breathe calmly.

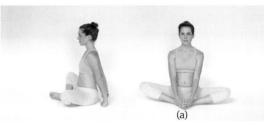

(a)

(a) For a variation, grasp your feet with both hands and keep bouncing your knees.

Training Focus: All movements involving knee and hip joints, many Yantras incorporating *tsokyil* position, in particular the 2nd and 3rd Tsigjongs, the Spider, the Lion, the Vulture, the Triangle, the Trident, and lotus position

9. KNEES TO THE CHEST

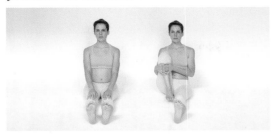

Sit with your legs straight in front. Inhale, then exhale while using both hands to pull one knee to your chest, keeping your foot suspended in the air in front of your perineum. Inhale as you stretch your leg back on the floor. Exhale and bring the other knee to your chest, continuing to alternate the sequence three to five times.

Training Focus: All movements involving knee and hip joints, in particular the Curved Knife, the Dove, and the Eagle

10. KNEES TO THE SIDE

Sitting with both legs in front of you, inhale, bringing one heel to your perineum with the opposite hand, and exhale calmly while gently pushing your knee toward the floor. Inhale, straightening the leg in front and bringing the other heel to your perineum, then exhale, gently pushing your other knee to the floor, repeating three to five times on each side.

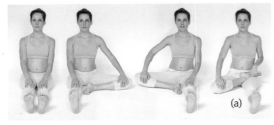

(a)

(a) In a variation, inhale, bringing your foot on top of your thigh at your groin, and gently bounce your knee up and down with

your corresponding hand while calmly exhaling. Inhale, straightening your leg in front and bringing your other foot to the top of your other thigh, then gently bounce your knee up and down with the corresponding hand while calmly exhaling. Repeat three to five times on each side.

Training Focus: All movements involving knee joints, in particular the Conch, the Curved Knife, and the Eagle

11. HIP AND KNEE RELAXER

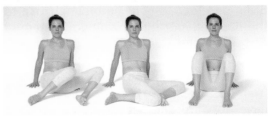

Sitting on the floor, raise your knees up by planting your feet about a foot's length in front of your buttocks and a hip width apart, leaning back slightly and supporting yourself with your hands behind your back. Inhale, straightening your back, then exhale, lowering both knees to one side, with one knee coming to the floor close to your other foot and your other knee opening wide. Keep the movement loose and relaxed. Inhale, lifting both knees up to the starting position. Exhale, lowering your knees to the other side, continuing to alternate for three to five repetitions.

Training Focus: All movements involving the knee and hip joints, in particular the Turtle and the Tiger

12. Knee to the Side Forward Bend

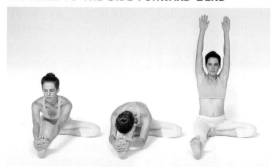

Start by sitting with your back straight and your legs stretched in front and parallel. Bring one foot to your perineum, close to the base of your thigh, with your knee on or toward the floor. Inhale, raising your arms straight over your head, keeping your spine straight. Exhale, bending forward from the base of your spine, moving your navel forward and allowing your spine to lengthen. Without forcing, try to bring your forehead toward the knee of your straight leg, wrapping your hands around your foot or ankle or just stretching toward your toes. Go only as far as you can with your back straight. Gradually bring your forehead closer to your knee and your fingers to or toward your toes, continuing to inhale and exhale. Switch sides and repeat, continuing to alternate the entire sequence three to five times.

Do this exercise only if it does not cause you to force or strain. Once you are sufficiently flexible, you can deepen the stretch by placing your foot on the top of the thigh at the groin.

Training Focus: All movements involving forward bending or the knee and hip joints, in particular the Conch, the Curved Knife, and the Eagle

13. Both Knees to the Side Forward Bend

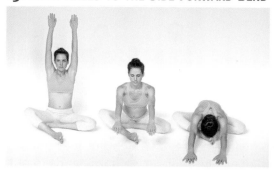

Sitting on the floor, place one foot at your perineum and the other two hand spans in front of your perineum, opening both knees outward and bringing them to or near the floor. Inhale, extending your arms straight above your head, and exhale, bending forward and bringing your forehead toward or to your front foot. Keep your arms stretched forward, if possible resting your hands on the floor. Stretch from the base of your spine and keep your back straight but not tense. Inhale, raising your arms back above your head, then exhale, bending forward. Repeat three to five times, then reverse the position of your legs and repeat again.

Training Focus: All movements involving forward bending or the knee and hip joints, in particular the Spider, the Lion, the Jewel, and lotus position

14. SOLES TOGETHER FORWARD BEND

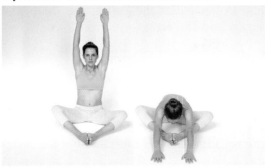

Bring the soles of your feet together two hand spans in front of your perineum, with your knees open to the sides and on or near the floor. Inhale, stretching your arms up. Exhale, bending forward from the base of your spine, and bring your forehead toward your extended feet. Keep your arms stretched out in front. You can also hold on to your feet to help lower your forehead more. Repeat the sequence three to five times.

Training Focus: All movements involving forward bending or the knee and hip joints, in particular the Trident, the Jewel, and lotus position

15. TURNING AND STRETCHING

This exercise is a particularly effective and comprehensive warm-up, and it helps you develop the correct sitting position. It is also highly useful for training for the lotus pose.

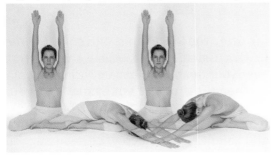

Sit on the floor with one leg bent in front with the heel at your perineum. Bend your other leg behind you, keeping the foot close to your buttocks without sitting on it. Inhaling, stretch your arms up and parallel. Turn from the root of your spine as you exhale, placing your forehead on the floor in front of one knee as you extend your arms to the floor. Inhaling, straighten your spine, and keeping your arms extended above your head, turn to the other side and bring your forehead in front of your other knee, extending your arms forward. Repeat three to five times. Reverse the position of your legs and repeat the sequence on the other side.

More than likely, you will find one side significantly easier than the other.

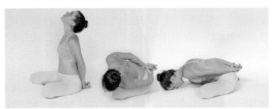

(a) Sitting in the same position, clasp your hands behind your back and circle over your knees, inhaling as you arch back and exhaling as you bring your forehead over one knee and then the other, circling three to five times in a continuous flow, sweeping your face near the floor and trying to keep your buttocks on the floor. Reverse the direction of the circling motion, then switch the position of your legs and repeat the same sequence on the other side.

Training Focus: Complete breathing in general, Nine Purification Breathings, all movements involving the spine, neck, arms, or knee and hip joints, in particular the Spider, the Triangle, the Dove, the Tiger, the Eagle, and lotus position

16. KNEE BEND

This exercise is best performed after doing the Turning and Stretching warm-up. Do not attempt it at the start of a warm-up session.

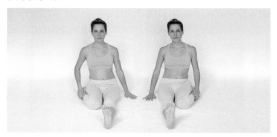

Sit with your legs in front and your back straight, your hands on the floor to your sides. Inhale smoothly and calmly, then exhale, leaning slightly to one side and using your hand as a support. At the same time, bend your other knee back and bring your foot to the side, your toes pointing backward close to your body as you place both buttocks on the floor. Inhale, stretching your leg in front again, then exhale and repeat the movement on the opposite side, continuously alternating sides three to five times.

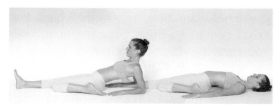

(a) Again bending one knee and pointing your foot back while you keep your other leg stretched, lean backward on your elbows. If you can, and if it is comfortable enough, lie on the floor and relax a moment, breathing calmly. Switch sides and repeat, continuing to alternate the entire sequence several times.

Training Focus: All movements involving the knee and hip joints or backward bending, in particular the Turtle, the Dove, the Tiger, and the Frog

17. CROSSED KNEE STRETCH

The next two exercises are important for training some fundamental movements to be performed as part of the main practice, in particular three of the Lungsangs. Ideally, one knee is directly over the other one.

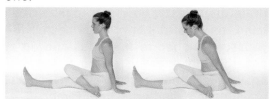

Sitting with one leg extended, cross your other leg over your knee, bending your foot back and placing it next to your hip. Place your palms on the floor behind you with your fingers pointing back. Inhale as you open your chest and fill your lungs. Bending forward over your thigh, exhale, then inhale as you move back to the upright position.

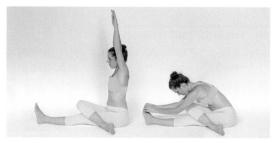

(a) After repeating this movement three to five times, inhale, raising your arms over your head, and exhale, bringing your forehead in front of your knee and your fingers to or toward the toes of your extended foot. Inhale and exhale smoothly and calmly. Try to keep your head aligned with your spine. Switch sides and repeat.

Training Focus: All movements involving the knee and hip joints, crossed knees, or forward bending, in particular the 3rd, 6th, and 8th Lungsangs, the Conch, and the Eagle

18. KNEE OVER KNEE

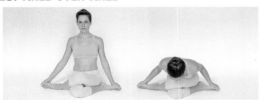

Sitting on the floor with your legs extended, bend one leg back under the knee of your other leg, then bend your upper leg back to the other side, coming to a position with one knee over the other, both buttocks on the floor. Place your hands on your feet. Keeping your spine straight and controlled, inhale, opening your chest, then exhale, bending forward over your knees in a movement starting at the base of your spine. Inhale, coming back to the starting position. Repeat three to five times, then reverse the position of your legs and repeat again.

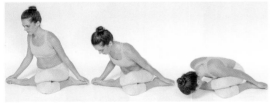

(a) In a modification incorporating a twist, exhaling, turn to the open side and bend over your lower thigh in a movement starting from the base of your spine. Inhaling, come back to the center, turn to the closed side, and bend over your upper thigh as you exhale. Repeat three to five times, then reverse the position of your legs and repeat again.

Training Focus: All movements involving the knee and hip joints, crossed knees, torsions, or forward bending, in particular the 3rd, 6th, and 8th Lungsangs, the Conch, the Curved Knife, and the Eagle

19. SIDE STRETCH

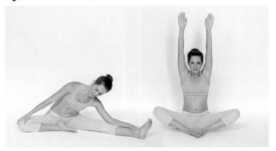

Sit with your back straight and your legs in front of you. Inhaling, raise your arms over your head and bring the soles of your feet together. Exhaling, bring your hands to your knees. Inhaling, raise your arms up. Exhaling, open one leg wide to the side and bend your torso sideways toward it as you bring the corresponding hand to or toward the outside of your extended foot while keeping the other hand on your bent knee. Inhaling, raise your arms over your head and bring the soles of your feet together again. Exhaling, open your other leg wide open to the side, reaching your hand to or toward your extended foot. Switch sides and repeat, continuing to alternate the entire sequence three to five times while calmly inhaling and exhaling.

Training Focus: All movements involving the spine, hip joints, or side stretching, in particular the Half-Moon and the Triangle

20. OPEN FORWARD STRETCH

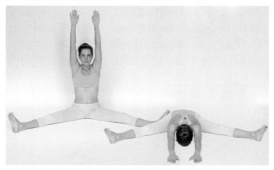

Seated with both legs wide open, inhale, raising your arms straight up. Exhale, bringing your hands to or toward the floor in front of you, reaching as far forward as you can while keeping your back straight. Bending from the hips and continuing to breathe, gradually lower your forehead closer to the floor, going only as far as you can without rounding your back. Do not force yourself at any time, just gently and steadily try to improve your range of movement.

Training Focus: All movements involving the spine, hip joints, or forward bending, in particular many concluding phases, the Half-Moon, the Triangle, the Trident, and the Tiger

21. GENTLE SPINE TWIST

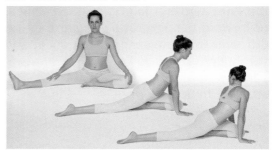

Begin seated on the floor with one leg extended out and the other bent with the foot at your perineum. Turn from the base of your spine toward your bent knee and place one hand on either side of the knee. Continue to turn in the same direction as you lift your buttocks and straighten your arms to look over your shoulder back at the foot of your extended leg. You will experience a gentle torsion of the spine and waist. Repeat on the other side for a total of three to five repetitions.

Training Focus: All movements involving torsion of the spine, in particular the Conch, the Half-Moon, and the Dove

22. TRANSITION TRAINING

The next exercise is important because it helps train the transition linking many of the sequences in Yantra Yoga. It is also highly effective for working on the leg joints. Coordinate the movement with your breathing, and use the momentum of the movement to help you roll onto your knees, progressing from one step to the next in a continuous sequence. If necessary, use a thin cushion or prop beneath your buttocks, and use your hands as a support to help you through the motions. Alternatively, you can come into the kneeling position by crossing your legs close to the pubis and rolling up onto your knees that way (as in the transition movement of the fourth Tsigjong).

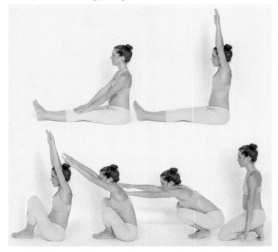

Sitting with your legs extended in front of you, inhale and raise your arms up. Exhale, bringing your arms horizontal in front of you as you roll forward onto your knees and sit back on your heels with your toes curled under and your arms along your sides.

Inhale, raising your arms over your head and coming up on your knees, keeping your toes curled under. Exhale, sitting back on your heels, bringing the tops of your feet flat on the floor and arms along your sides. Inhale, rising back up onto your knees with your arms above your head, the tops of your feet still flat on the floor. Exhale, curling your toes under, rolling onto the soles of your feet and sitting on your buttocks with your arms along your sides. Inhale, extending your legs in front of you while raising your arms parallel above your head. Exhale, bringing your hands to your knees or bending forward to bring your fingers to your toes and forehead to your knees. Repeat the entire sequence three to five times.

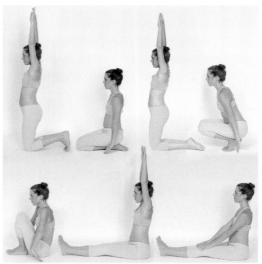

Training Focus: All movements involving the hip and knee joints, in particular many transition movements, the 4th Tsigjong, the 4th Lungsang, the Turtle, the Dagger, and the Vulture

Face-Up Warm-Ups

The next warm-ups are done lying on your back. They are simple but highly effective exercises for the lower spine in particular.

23. KNEE TO CHEST

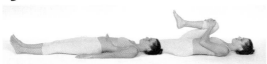

Lying on your back, exhale and bring one knee to your chest, clasping it with both hands. Then inhale, stretching your leg along the floor again, keeping it well extended and straight. Exhale, bringing your other knee to your chest, then inhale as you extend your leg back along the floor. Switch sides and repeat, continuing to alternate the entire sequence three to five times.

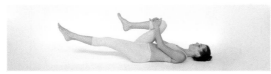

(a) Repeat the same exercise, but keep your extended leg just above the floor when you bring your knee to your chest.

With each exhalation, pull your knee increasingly closer to your chest.

Training Focus: All movements involving the knee and hip joints, hamstrings, or lower back

24. PERPENDICULAR LEG STRETCH

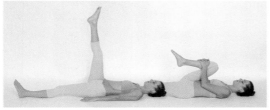

Lying on your back, inhale and extend one

leg straight up. Exhale, bending the leg and bringing your knee to your chest with both hands. Inhale, extending your leg straight up, then exhale as you lower the leg to the floor. Switch sides and repeat, continuing to alternate the entire sequence three to five times.

Training Focus: All movements involving the knee and hip joints, hamstrings, or lower back, in particular the Flame and the Plow

25. LEG SWEEP

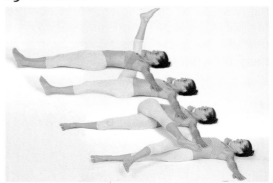

Lying on your back with your arms stretched out to the sides, inhale and extend one leg straight up. Then exhale and cross the leg over to the other side of your body, bringing your toes toward the floor around hip height. Skimming the floor with your toes, sweep your upper leg in a circle over the ankle of the leg that is on the floor, and come back to starting position with both legs stretched out. Keep your shoulders on the floor throughout the exercise. Switch sides and repeat, continuing to alternate the entire sequence three to five times.

Training Focus: All movements involving the knee and hip joints, in particular the Half-Moon and the Eagle

26. HIP RELEASER

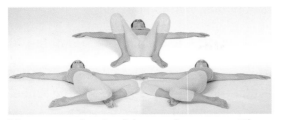

Lie on your back with your knees up. Place your feet at the base of your buttocks, with your toes pointing out to the sides at a wide angle. Your arms are extended out to the sides at shoulder level. Inhale deeply and relax. Exhale and roll both knees over to one side as far as they will go without forcing them, keeping your shoulders on the floor. Inhale, coming back to the center. Exhale, rolling your knees to the other side. Repeat three to five times, breathing calmly and coordinating the stretch with the breathing.

Training Focus: All movements involving the knee and hip joints or the lower back, in particular the Turtle and the Tiger

27. SUPINE TWIST

This exercise is a simple and safe torsion that is especially effective for keeping the back healthy.

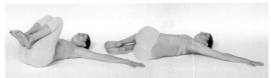

Lying on your back, bring your knees to your chest, then roll onto one side, keeping your knees and your feet close together. Inhaling, open and stretch your top arm to the other side, keeping your shoulders and your knees on the floor. Look straight up and breathe deeply and smoothly, relaxing in the pose. Roll onto the other side

and repeat, continuing to alternate three to five times.

(a) In a variation, roll onto one side and place your top knee on the floor in front of your bottom knee. Place your lower hand on your top knee to keep it on the floor, then stretch your other arm out to the side while keeping your shoulders firmly on the floor. Look straight up and breathe deeply and smoothly. Roll onto the other side and repeat, continuing to alternate three to five times.

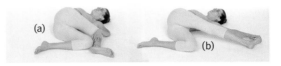

(b) For yet another variation, extend your upper leg over your bent knee, stretching it as straight as possible and holding onto your toes with your lower hand. Roll onto the other side and repeat, continuing to alternate three to five times.

If it is difficult to hold onto your toes, you can use a scarf, towel, or yoga belt around your foot to help you stretch your leg.

Training Focus: All Yantras involving torsions, in particular the 3rd, 6th, and 8th Lungsangs, the Conch, the Curved Knife, and the Eagle

28. HIP OPENER

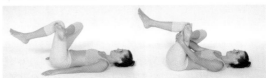

Lie on your back with your heels close to your buttocks and your arms along your sides. Place one ankle on top of your thigh above the knee and bring the knee up

toward your chest, wrapping your hands around the front of the knee or the back of your thigh and pulling it gently closer toward your chest. Inhale and exhale calmly. Switch sides and repeat the sequence three to five times.

Training Focus: All movements involving knee and hip joints, in particular the Plow, the Curved Knife, the Dagger, and lotus position

29. BRIDGE

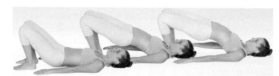

Lie on your back with your heels close to your buttocks and your arms to your sides. Inhaling, raise your hips in the air as you gently lift your lower back off the floor, then exhale, rolling your spine back to the floor. Repeat the sequence three to five times, arching a little more with each new inhalation, but without forcing, consciously coordinating the continuous flow of the movement of your body with the flow of your breath. Exhale gently and rest a moment on the floor.

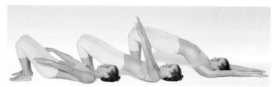

(a) Repeat the exercise, but this time stretch your arms straight above your head as you inhale and arch your back. Exhaling, bring your arms forward to come back to the floor near your feet while you gradually roll your spine to the floor, co-

ordinating movement and breathing in a continuous, harmonious flow.

Training Focus: Complete breathing in general, Nine Purification Breathings, all movements involving back bending, in particular the Camel, the Bow, and the Wheel

30. SPINE ROLL

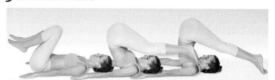

Lying on your back, exhale and bring your knees toward your chest, rolling onto your shoulders as you extend your legs and bring your feet toward the floor above your head, gently and without forcing. You can practice this warm-up with the aid of a chair or cushions until you can extend your feet toward the floor. Keep your arms extended on the floor along your sides. Inhaling, roll forward and bring your feet back to the floor in front of you. Keep your spine straight and your knees together. Repeat three to five times.

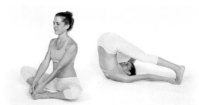

(a) In a variation, start sitting upright with the soles of your feet together and your knees open to the side. Grab your toes and inhale as you straighten your back. Exhale, rolling back, still holding your toes, to bring your legs wide open above your head. Inhale and roll forward to the starting position. Repeat three to five times.

Training Focus: All movements actively involving the spine, in particular the Flame, the Plow, the Triangle, and the Trident

Face-Down Warm-Ups

The next exercises are done in a prone position. They mainly benefit the spine and the leg joints.

31. CAT

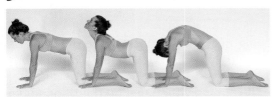

Come to your hands and knees with your knees shoulder-width apart and your hands underneath your shoulders, keeping your arms straight. Your palms and the tops of your feet are flat on the floor. Inhale, lowering your navel while bringing your pelvis parallel to the floor and arching your head back. Exhale, bringing your pelvis perpendicular to the floor, curving your back upward like a cat, and bringing your head between your arms and your chin to your chest. Repeat the sequence three to five times.

It is important not to block the breathing but let it flow freely with the rhythm of the movement.

Training Focus: Complete breathing in general, Nine Purification Breathings, all movements involving the spine, neck, or back bending, in particular the Camel, the Bow, and the Wheel

32. LOCUST TRAINING

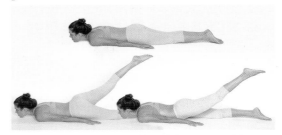

Lie on your stomach with your chin on the floor and your arms along your sides. Inhaling, raise one leg up, keeping it controlled and straight with your foot pointed. Try to not to bend your knees or open and rotate your hip. Exhaling, lower your leg back to the floor. Switch to the other side and repeat, continuing to alternate three to five times.

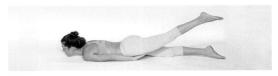

(a) For an easier variation, put your hands under your thighs, palms up.

Training Focus: All movements involving back bending, in particular the Bow, the Locust, and the Wheel

33. SNAKE TRAINING

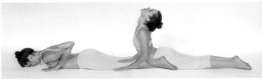

Lie on your stomach with your forehead on the floor and your hands at chest level. Inhaling, slowly raise your torso up and arch your head back, exhaling, bring your forehead to the floor. Keep your movements slow and coordinated. Repeat three to five times.

Training Focus: All movements involving back bending, in particular the Camel, the Dog, the Snake, the Bow, and the Dove

34. SNAKE TRAINING II

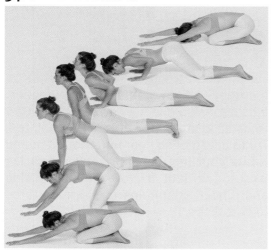

Lie on your stomach with your forehead on the floor and your arms along your sides. Inhale and bring your palms alongside your chest. Keeping your palms on the floor and your arms stretched in front of you, raise your torso up and sit back on your heels as you exhale. Still keeping your palms on the floor, inhale, slide your torso forward close to the floor, then arch your upper body back while trying to keep your lower pubis on the floor. Exhaling, bring your buttocks back to your heels and your forehead to the floor between your arms. Continuing the flow of the breathing and the movement, inhale, sliding forward and arching back as before, always keeping your palms in the same position in front of you. Exhale, sitting on your heels with your arms stretched forward and your forehead to the floor. Repeat three to five times.

Training Focus: All movements involving back bending, in particular the Camel, the

Snake, the Dog, the Bow, the Dove, and the Wheel

35. SOLES TOGETHER HIP OPENER
This exercise is particularly effective for training the lotus position.

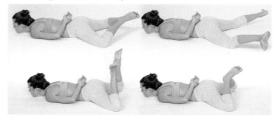

Lying on your stomach with your chin on the floor, spread your knees open while placing the soles of your feet together and keeping your navel on the floor. Clasp your hands behind your back and gradually bring your feet to the floor without separating them. Inhale, opening your legs wide, and exhale, joining your feet and bringing them back toward the floor. Repeat three to five times.

Training Focus: Complete breathing in general, Nine Purification Breathings, all movements involving hip joints, in particular the Vulture and lotus position

36. DOG TRAINING

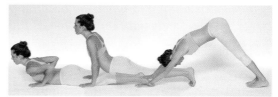

Lie on your stomach with your forehead on the floor and your hands at chest level, the tops of your feet on the floor. Inhaling, raise your head up and arch your upper body back. Exhaling, curl your toes under and counterarch your back as you bring your buttocks into the air, keeping your

arms and legs straight. Your head stays between your extended arms while the palms of your hands and the soles of your feet are firmly on the floor, if possible. If it is too difficult, try to keep your heels as close to the floor as you can. Inhaling, lower your pelvis and your navel toward the floor, but keep your thighs parallel to the floor and your arms straight as you arch your spine and your head. Exhale, bringing your buttocks back into the air as you lower your heels back toward the floor. Repeat three to five times, breathing calmly and smoothly with the flow of the movement.

Training Focus: All movements involving back bending, in particular the Dog and the Tiger

Neck and Shoulder Opening Warm-Ups

37. NECK ROLL
This exercise helps train the flexibility of the neck. Like all of the warm-ups, it should be done calmly and with attention, without forcing the movement or the breathing.

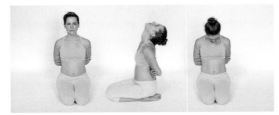

Sitting on your heels, bring your arms behind your back and grab your forearms above the elbows or at the wrists. Inhale, arching your head back by stretching your chin up, then exhale, bringing your chin toward your chest, repeating three or five times.

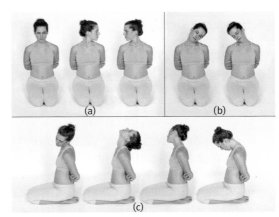

(a)   (b)

(c)

(a) Then inhale to the center and exhale, turning your head gently but fully to the side. Inhale, moving your head back to the center, and exhale, turning to the other side. Repeat three or five times.

(b) Now exhale, moving one ear toward your shoulder. Inhale, raising your head back to the center, then exhale, bringing your other ear toward your other shoulder. Repeat three or five times.

(c) Finally, rotate your head, inhaling while arching your neck back and exhaling, rotating to the front. First turn in one direction three to five times, then turn in the other direction.

Training Focus: All movements involving the neck or back bending, in particular the 6th Lungsang, the Camel, the Conch, the Snake, the Bow, the Dove, and the Wheel

38. Shoulder Opener

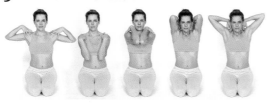

Sitting on your heels, bring your hands to the top of your shoulders and join your elbows in front of your chest. Inhaling, open your elbows up and back as you rotate your shoulders. Exhaling, bring your elbows down in a circular direction and join them in front again. Then rotate your elbows in the opposite direction. Repeat in each direction three to five times.

Training Focus: All movements involving the shoulders

39. Shoulder and Chest Opener

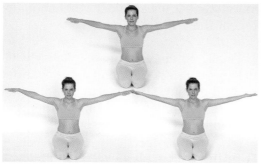

Sitting on your heels with your arms open wide and your palms up, exhale, rotating your shoulders and closing them to the front as you turn your palms to face the floor. Inhaling, rotate your shoulders back and open as you turn your hands the other way, bringing the palms face up again. Repeat the sequence three to five times.

Here, as in the previous exercise, it is important to breathe with intent and energy.

Training Focus: Complete breathing in general, Nine Purification Breathings, all movements actively involving the arms and chest, in particular the 5th Tsigjong, the Curved Knife, and the Bow

40. Shoulder Opener II

Sitting on your heels, raise one arm up and bring your hand toward your shoulder blade. With your other hand, grab the elbow of that arm behind your head and pull it toward your opposite shoulder, stretching the side of your arm and torso. Repeat several times on each side.

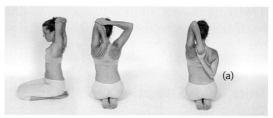

(a)

(a) Again raise one arm and bring your hand to your shoulder blade, but this time reach behind and up your back with your other hand and try to hook the fingers of both hands together in an S-shape. If you cannot reach, either stretch as far as possible while keeping your spine straight, or use a scarf or belt as a bridge. Switch to the other side, then repeat the sequence three to five times.

If you do this exercise regularly, your range will improve over time. Always breathe in an easy and relaxed way.

Training Focus: All movements involving the shoulders

41. ARM STRETCH

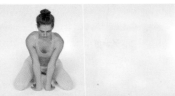

Sitting on your heels with your knees open, place your palms between your knees with your fingers pointing toward your perineum to stretch your arms. Relax and breathe calmly and smoothly, keeping your back straight and your shoulders open as you stretch.

Training Focus: All movements actively involving the arms and wrists, in particular the Peacock

Appendix 2
Suggested Practice Routines

THE ROUTINES SUGGESTED here are just a general guideline. Depending on your personal pace, the shortest can take anywhere between five and eight minutes and the longest well over an hour. Although of course the longer sessions bring the most benefit, even the very shortest, done regularly and with attention, will have a noticeably positive effect on your vital energy and well-being.

ANYTIME QUICK ROUTINE
approximately 7 minutes
Warm-Up 4 and 4a (Shaking the Feet): three repetitions each
Warm-Up 5 (Swinging the Lower Legs): three repetitions
Warm-Up 10 (Knees to the Side): three repetitions
Three-exhalation version of Nine Purification Breathings
    (see the chapter on Nine Purification Breathings)
Rhythmic Breathing 4–4–4: three rounds

QUICK TUNE-UP ROUTINE
approximately 12 minutes
Warm-Up 4 and 4a (Shaking the Feet): five repetitions each
Warm-Up 5 (Swinging the Lower Legs): five repetitions
Warm-Up 31 (Cat): five repetitions
Three-exhalation version of Nine Purification Breathings
    (see the chapter on Nine Purification Breathings)
Eight Lungsang Movements (short version, see below)
Rhythmic Breathing 4–4–4: six rounds
Three fast exhalations or one Vajra Wave plus brief relaxation
    (see chapter on the Vajra Wave)

BASIC ROUTINE
approximately 18 minutes
Warm-Up 4 and 4a (Shaking the Feet): five repetitions each
Warm-Up 5 (Swinging the Lower Legs): five repetitions
Warm-Up 27, 27a, and 27b (Supine Twist): one repetition each
Warm-Up 34 (Snake Training II): three repetitions
Warm-Up 37, 37a, 37b, 37c (Neck Roll): three repetitions each
Three-exhalation version of Nine Purification Breathings
   (see chapter on the Nine Purification Breathings)
Eight Lungsang Movements (full version, see below)
Rhythmic Breathing 4–4–4: six rounds
Seven fast exhalations or one Vajra Wave plus relaxation
   (see chapter on the Vajra Wave)

SHORT ROUTINE
approximately 30 minutes
Warm-Up 4 and 4a (Shaking the Feet): five repetitions each
Warm-Up 8 and 8a (Butterfly)
Warm-Up 6 (Rotating the Legs): three repetitions each side
Warm-Up 24 (Perpendicular Leg Stretch): three repetitions each side
Warm-Up 26 (Hip Releaser): three repetitions
Warm-Up 31 (Cat): five repetitions
Nine Purification Breathings
Five Tsigjong Movements (short version, see below)
Eight Lungsang Movements (short version, see below)
First Series of Yantras (or five assorted Yantras in con-
   secutive order of holds; short version, see below)
Rhythmic Breathing 4–4–4 and 4–6–6: three rounds each
Seven fast exhalations or three Vajra Waves plus relaxation
   (see chapter on the Vajra Wave)

MEDIUM ROUTINE
approximately 45 minutes
Warm-Up 4 and 4a (Shaking the Feet): five repetitions each
Warm-Up 8 and 8a (Butterfly)
Warm-Up 6 (Rotating the Legs): three repetitions each side
Warm-Up 27, 27a, and 27b (Supine Twist): one repetition each
Warm-Up 28 (Hip Opener)
Warm-Up 29a (Bridge)
Warm-Up 37, 37a, 37b, 37c (Neck Roll): three repetitions each
Nine Purification Breathings
Five Tsigjong Movements (short version, see below)
Eight Lungsang Movements (full version, see below)

Five Tsadul Movements (short version, see below)
First Series of Yantras (short version, see below)
Second Series of Yantras (short version, see below)
Rhythmic Breathing 4–4–4 and 4–6–6: three rounds each
Seven fast exhalations or three Vajra Waves plus relaxation
  (see chapter on the Vajra Wave)

FULL ROUTINE
approximately 60 minutes
Ten to fifteen minutes of warm-ups of your choice
  (see above and Appendix 1 for suggestions)
Nine Purification Breathings
Five Tsigjong Movements (full version, see below)
Eight Lungsang Movements (full version, see below)
Tsadul Breathing
Five Tsadul Movements (full version, see below)
Brief relaxation
One full series of Yantras (or five assorted Yantras in con-
  secutive order of holds; full version, see below)
Rhythmic Breathing 4–4–4, 4–6–4, and 4–6–6: three rounds each
Seven fast exhalations or three Vajra Waves plus relaxation
  (see chapter on the Vajra Wave)

EXTENDED ROUTINE
approximately 80 minutes
Fifteen to twenty minutes of warm-ups of your choice
  (see above and Appendix 1 for suggestions)
Nine Purification Breathings
Five Tsigjong Movements (full version, see below)
Eight Lungsang Movements (full version, see below)
Tsadul Breathing
Five Tsadul Movements (full version, see below)
Brief relaxation
Two full series of Yantras (or two series of assorted Yantras
  in consecutive order of holds; full version, see below)
Rhythmic Breathing 4–4–4, 4–6–4, and 4–6–6: five rounds each
Three Vajra Waves plus relaxation

Short and Full Versions of Tsigjongs, Lungsangs, Tsaduls, and Yantras

SHORT VERSION OF FIVE TSIGJONG MOVEMENTS
1st Tsigjong: three repetitions
2nd Tsigjong: three repetitions each phase
3rd Tsigjong: three repetitions each side, skip third phase
4th Tsigjong: one repetition
5th Tsigjong: three repetitions

FULL VERSION OF FIVE TSIGJONG MOVEMENTS
1st Tsigjong: seven repetitions
2nd Tsigjong: three repetitions each phase
3rd Tsigjong: three repetitions each phase
4th Tsigjong: three repetitions
5th Tsigjong: seven repetitions

SHORT VERSION OF EIGHT LUNGSANG MOVEMENTS
1st Lungsang: one repetition
2nd Lungsang: all three phases
3rd Lungsang: both sides
4th Lungsang: one repetition
5th Lungsang: one repetition
6th Lungsang: both sides
7th Lungsang: one repetition
8th Lungsang: both sides

FULL VERSION OF EIGHT LUNGSANG MOVEMENTS
1st Lungsang: three repetitions
2nd Lungsang: all three phases
3rd Lungsang: both sides
4th Lungsang: three repetitions
5th Lungsang: three repetitions
6th Lungsang: both sides
7th Lungsang: three repetitions
8th Lungsang: both sides

SHORT VERSION OF FIVE TSADUL MOVEMENTS
1st Tsadul: one repetition
2nd Tsadul: both sides
3rd Tsadul: one repetition
4th Tsadul: one repetition
5th Tsadul: one repetition

Long Version of Five Tsadul Movements

1st Tsadul: three repetitions
2nd Tsadul: both sides
3rd Tsadul: three repetitions
4th Tsadul: three repetitions
5th Tsadul: three repetitions

Short Version of Each of the Five Series of Yantras

1st Yantra: one repetition
2nd Yantra: both sides
3rd Yantra: one repetition
4th Yantra: one repetition
5th Yantra: one repetition

Full Version of Each of the Five Series of Yantras

1st Yantra: three repetitions
2nd Yantra: both sides
3rd Yantra: three repetitions
4th Yantra: three repetitions
5th Yantra: three repetitions

Appendix 3
Yantra Yoga and Tibetan Medicine

By Phuntsog Wangmo, Tibetan doctor and Academic Director of the Shang Shung Institute School of Tibetan Medicine

EVERYTHING IN THE universe is interdependent. The external world, the environment, and the internal world of sentient beings are also interdependent and support and benefit each other. For example, if human beings take care of the land, it nourishes and sustains them. In the same way, the various forms of knowledge, such as astrology, medicine, dharma or inner knowledge, and yoga, are all interdependent and support each other. But in the case of Tibetan yoga and Tibetan medicine, the link is particularly strong. While the anatomy of the physical body is based on medical principles, yoga explains how the channels are developed, how they are connected, and how energy flows through them.

When we study disease in Tibetan medicine, we study the theory of the five elements, earth, water, fire, air, and space, each with its own function, nature, and quality. Earth is related to form, fire to digestion, water to making things smooth, air to circulation and keeping things flowing, and space to making room for development. Emotionally, earth and water are related to calmness and stability, fire is related to determination and mental sharpness, and air to thoughts. Sickness arises when the five elements are imbalanced, when one or more elements are excessive, deficient, or disturbed. At this point, the aim of treatment is to bring things back into balance.

Wind is involved with circulation. Circulation implies that there is a path to go on, and Yantra Yoga mainly works with channels and wind. Both Tibetan medicine and yoga compare the channels to pathways. Various visible fluids and invisible energies travel on these pathways, propelled by wind, the energy that pushes or accompanies them. Another metaphor to illustrate these three aspects is that the

245

channels are like roads, the fluids or energies traveling in them are passengers, and wind is the vehicle that conveys them. The channels constitute the basis of the physical body. They are formed during the fourth week of fetal development, starting with three major channels and followed by the remaining twenty-one thousand channels that traverse the body. These channels can be considered like a net that supports the body. Because it harmonizes the flow of energy in the channels, doing yoga can help balance the body and counteract illness. When we are not sick, yoga can help us maintain good health.

Tibetan medicine distinguishes five types of wind (*lung* in Tibetan and *prana* in Sanskrit). The first is the life-sustaining wind, located at the crown chakra and traveling downward through the throat to the chest. It governs the functions of swallowing, inhaling, burping, sneezing, and speech. The second is the ascending wind, located in the chest and moving upward through the throat. It controls the function of speech, gives us strength and determination, defines our complexion, and helps clarify memory. The third, called the pervasive wind, is located in the heart. It travels throughout the body and keeps things circulating. Most actions or movements of the body are connected with this wind. The fourth, the fire-accompanying wind, is located in the lower digestive system. It moves through all the digestive organs and helps us digest food, separating the pure from the impure parts of food. The fifth is the downward-clearing wind, located in the sacral or pelvic area. Its pathway is in the large intestine and reproductive organs, and it plays a role in the elimination of feces and urine as well as the production and release of reproductive fluids. It keeps things clean and opens and closes the orifices as necessary.

When the body is dysfunctional, one of these winds is invariably involved. For example, if you have difficulty inhaling or swallowing food, the life-sustaining wind is not working. If you are not able to speak or your voice is shaky, the ascending wind is imbalanced. When circulation is poor, the pervasive wind is disordered. If the digestive system is weak and causing organ disease, the fire-accompanying wind is dysfunctional. Constipation, miscarriage, delayed labor, and premature ejaculation can all be related to a malfunctioning of the descending wind. Once one of the five winds is imbalanced, particular symptoms or qualities will manifest that correspond with its specific nature. The nature of wind is light, rough, cold, hard, unstable, or subtle. The characteristics of wind disorders also commonly manifest as insomnia or mental instability.

Yantra Yoga mainly helps balance our health through breathing and movement. Done correctly, it can remove blockages of energy. Fresh breath is brought into the body through the breath and impure energy or air is breathed out. The movements, breathing, and holds in Yantra Yoga are all done with the express purpose of opening and restoring the channels. Specific movements are combined with specific breathing techniques consisting of inhalation, holds, and exhalation that correspond with certain channels and parts of the body, and they function to clean and restore these parts.

These yoga techniques benefit the digestive heat and help heal and balance all the internal organs, kidney function, and each of the five winds. They help clear the memory, mobilize the joints, move excess liquid out of the body, and tighten the muscles. Once all the channels are harmonized, whatever needs to move in the body travels in its proper place, and this in turn calms the mind. This is why we say yoga, and especially Yantra Yoga, is the best medicine to treat physical and mental disease and also the best prevention for physical and mental illness.

Glossary of Terms

asana: Sanskrit term for body position or posture. The literal meaning is "to sit," "to abide," and "to be present." Commonly used in Indian yoga traditions to refer to the individual poses adopted in practice.

ascending prana: Also called ascending wind; one of the five winds or pranas. Circulates throughout the tongue, nose, and throat and into the channels of the senses. Its function is to regulate speech, memory, and mental functions in general. It gives strength and courage. See *pranas, five* for a list of all five pranas.

Ati Yoga: See *Dzogchen*.

Ayurveda: The traditional medical system of India, generally considered to have originated some five thousand years ago. Numerous parallels exist between Ayurveda and Tibetan medicine, notably the identification of three humors, energies, or *doshas* (a Sanskrit term that literally means "fault" or "deficiency") and the concept that their balance or imbalance determines good or poor health. Ayurveda applies numerous modalities of treatment, ranging from the use of herbal, mineral, and animal substances to diet and massage. See also *energies, three* and *Tibetan traditional medicine*.

bile energy: In Tibetan medicine, one of the three humors or energies that form the basis for the functioning of the human body. Bile energy predominantly refers to the heat present in all parts of the body as the base of the life force. Residing in the digestive tract, liver, gallbladder, heart, blood, eyes, and skin, it has various functions. In particular, it regenerates all the bodily constituents and the blood. Strength and courage in achieving personal aims, analytical judgment, a good complexion, good eyesight, digestive heat, proper metabolism, and bodily temperature all depend on bile energy. The Tibetan term for bile energy is *tripa*. Ayurveda uses the Sanskrit word *pitta*. See also *energies, three*.

channels, subtle: See *nadis*.

complete breathing: Fundamental quality of breathing in Yantra Yoga. Inhaling through the nostrils, we fill the lungs gradually from the bottom to the top, as if filling a vase with water. Exhaling through the nostrils, we empty the top of the lungs first and the lower part of the lungs last.

cubit: Unit of measurement based on the length of the forearm from the elbow to the tip of the middle finger, usually equivalent to about eighteen inches. Two cubits are the distance from one elbow to the other when the fingertips are joined horizontally in front of the chest.

direct breathing: Term used in Yantra Yoga to describe smooth and calm breathing, free of any blockage or constriction in the throat. With the exception of two pranayamas, all of the exercises in this book use direct breathing for both the inhalations and exhalations. See also *indirect breathing.*

downward-clearing prana: Also called downward-clearing wind; one of the five winds or pranas. Located in the pelvic region, it circulates in the lower organs and regulates the production and emission of semen and menstrual fluids, the expulsion of feces and urine, and the process of childbirth. See *pranas, five* for a list of all five pranas.

Dzogchen: The Tibetan word *Dzogchen* means "total" *(chen)* "perfection" *(dzog),* the real condition of each individual. It refers to the self-perfected state, the potentiality of our real nature. The method for acquiring knowledge of Dzogchen and discovering our real condition is called Dzogchen teaching. It is not a philosophical theory created by intellectual analysis but rather a direct experience. Knowledge of Dzogchen goes back to ancient times. In our era it was transmitted for the first time by a master called Garab Dorje a few centuries after Shakyamuni Buddha.

elements, five: According to Tibetan medicine and many other classical philosophies, the universe is made of up four elements: earth, water, fire, and air. Interacting in the dimension of space, the element that is the base for all other elements, these four produce the entire macrocosm of the universe and the microcosm of beings. In the Tibetan view of the physical body, the earth element corresponds to the flesh and bones; the water element to blood, lymph, and serum; the fire element to bodily heat; the air element to respiration; and the space element to the functions of the mind. Earth is related to form, water to making things smooth, fire to digestion, air to circulation and keeping things flowing, and space to making room for development. Emotionally, earth and water are related to calmness and stability, fire is related to determination and mental sharpness, and air to thoughts.

Sickness arises when the five elements are imbalanced—when one or more elements are excessive, deficient, or disturbed. The aim of treatment, and of practices such as Yantra Yoga, is to bring things back into balance.

energies, three: In Tibetan medicine, the three humors or energies are known as wind, bile, and phlegm. Wind, or prana, has the mobile quality of the air element. Bile has the hot quality of the fire element. Phlegm has the solid and stable qualities of the earth element and the moist and wet qualities of the water element. The three energies are the bases for the formation, life, and destruction of the human body and also determine our psychophysical constitution. Their equivalents in Ayurvedic medicine are *vata, pitta,* and *kapha.* See also *wind energy, bile energy,* and *phlegm energy.*

energy channels: See *nadis.*

fire-accompanying prana: Also called fire-accompanying wind; one of the five winds or pranas. Resides in the stomach and bowels and regulates digestive functions, the separation of nutrients from waste, and the assimilation of nutrients. See *pranas, five* for a list of all five pranas.

hollow organs, six: Term used in Tibetan traditional medicine. Specifically refers to the stomach, small intestine, large intestine, gall bladder, urinary bladder, and seminal vesicles or ovaries.

humors, three: See *energies, three.*

indirect breathing: Yantra Yoga uses the term *indirect breathing* to refer to a deliberately constricted method of breathing that is generally only used in pranayama exercises such as the Tsadul pranayama and the more advanced stages of Rhythmic Breathing. When we breathe indirectly, our glottis is constricted and the breathing produces a distinct sound. For a practical demonstration of indirect breathing, refer to the Tsadul Breathing exercise in the section on the five Tsadul movements.

life-sustaining prana: Also called life-sustaining wind. One of the five winds or pranas; moves within the head and thorax and in the channels of the sense organs. It regulates the functions of breathing, swallowing, sneezing, coughing, and so on. It gives clarity to the mind and the sense organs. Its malfunctioning can cause depressive syndrome and anxiety, among other conditions. See *pranas, five* for a list of all five pranas.

Lungsang: Literally "purifying the prana," the second of three preliminary groups in the practice of Yantra Yoga. It consists of eight interconnected exercises featuring different types of holds that purify the prana. The eight Lungsangs have the very specific goal of training and developing four different ways of inhaling and exhaling and especially four different ways of holding the breath.

mahasiddha: Sanskrit term literally meaning "great" *(maha)* "adept" *(siddha*; also meaning one who has attained the highest purpose, accomplished one). Humkara, the master who transmitted Yantra Yoga to Padmasambhava, was a *mahasiddha.*

nadis: Sanskrit term for physical and subtle channels. The literal meaning of *nadi* is "a river" or "a channel" through which something flows. According to all major systems of traditional Asian medicine—Indian, Chinese, and Tibetan—the prana, chi, *lung,* or life force flows through a network of subtle channels traversing the body. The Tibetan term *tsa* carries meanings including channel, passageway, root, and cause and refers to both physical channels like nerves, veins, and arteries and subtle and immaterial nadis or energy channels.

naljor: Tibetan term roughly equivalent to the Sanskrit word *yoga.* However, while *yoga* means "union," *naljor,* literally "arriving at" or "merging with" *(jor)* our "real state" *(nal),* more specifically refers to possessing the real knowledge of our spontaneously natural condition and being concretely in that knowledge.

organs: See *hollow organs* and *solid organs.*

pervasive prana: Also called pervasive wind; one of the five winds or pranas. Circulates throughout the body, mainly through the blood vessels and sensory nerves. It presides over blood circulation, hormonal secretions, the development of the body, joint movement, and proper functioning of the orifices. See *pranas, five* for a list of all five pranas.

phlegm energy: In Tibetan medicine, one of the three humors or energies that form the basis for the functioning of the human body. Represents primarily the humid and wet components of the organism, which have a cool nature. Residing in the head, tongue, salivary glands, spleen, pancreas, chest, stomach, kidneys, bladder, and joints, phlegm energy has various functions; in particular it maintains the moisture the body needs and produces gastric juices. Mental stability, the sense of satisfaction from sense perceptions, the experience of taste, the process of digesting food, and ease in movements and sleep all depend on phlegm energy. The Tibetan term for phlegm energy is *peken.* Ayurveda uses the Sanskrit word *kapha.* See also *energies, three.*

prana: Sanskrit term referring to both our physical breath and the essence of life itself, our energy, power, life force. The Tibetan term, *lung,* can also refer to the wind element or wind energy.

pranas, five: Also known as the five winds; five types of wind energy circulating in the body and controlling specific bodily functions. The five pranas are life-sustaining prana, ascending prana, pervasive prana, fire-accompanying prana, and downward-clearing prana. See also entries for each of the five pranas.

pranayama: Sanskrit term for breathing exercises, literally meaning "to control" *(yama)* the "breath" or "life force" *(prana)*. An alternate interpretation is that the word breaks down into *prana* and *ayama* ("extension"), and hence refers to the extension or expansion of the breath. Aside from making our respiration more calm and complete and hence relaxing the body and the mind, pranayama exercises help us strengthen and harmonize our life force by reactivating the correct circulation of prana in the channels. Pranayama is also a powerful tool for controlling our mind and emotions and must not be taken lightly. It is best to receive instruction directly from a teacher. We have deliberately presented only a few basic breathing exercises in this book.

solid organs, five: Term used in Tibetan traditional medicine; refers to the heart, lungs, liver, spleen, and kidneys.

span: Generally, the distance from the end of the thumb to the end of the little finger of a spread hand. Tibetans measure roughly the same distance from the end of the outstretched thumb to the end of the outstretched middle finger.

Tibetan traditional medicine: A practice of medicine that evolved over several thousand years, dating back to the pre-Buddhist Bön era in Tibet. Over time, it absorbed influences from Ayurveda, traditional Chinese, Byzantine, and Persian medicine, as well as from nearby countries like Nepal. Tibetan traditional medicine centers on the principle that the functioning of the human body is determined by the interaction of the three humors or energies: wind, bile, and phlegm. It views illnesses as the result of imbalances of the humors, among other factors, as a consequence of emotions such as ignorance, greed, and anger. Modes of treatment range from dietary and behavioral changes, including the introduction of appropriate physical exercise such as Yantra Yoga, to the administration of medicines and the application of external therapies.

Tsadul: Literally, "controlling the channels"; the third of three preliminary groups in the practice of Yantra Yoga. It consists of one pranayama and five vigorous exercises that help open and control the physical and energetic channels.

Tsigjong: Tibetan term that literally means "loosening the joints"; the first of three preliminary groups in the practice of Yantra Yoga. It consists of five exercises designed to warm up the body by loosening the joints.

tsokyil: A basic sitting posture used frequently in Yantra Yoga. The soles of the feet are joined about one or two hand-widths in front of the perineum, with the hands generally on the knees. Many Yantras (particularly in the third series) and some of the preliminary movements start in this pose. Warm-Up 8 (Butterfly) is particularly effective for practicing this pose.

vajra: The Sanskrit word *vajra*, literally "the hard one" or "the mighty one," is rich in meanings, including "indestructible," "diamond," and "thunderbolt." The term is used in Vajrayana Buddhism to refer to the true primordial nature of every living being, beyond birth and death. The Tibetan equivalent, *dorje,* literally means "the lord of stones." Vajra or dorje is also the name of a ritual instrument symbolizing the immutable, indestructible quality of the state of absolute reality.

vajra fist: A way to make a fist that is frequently employed in Yantra Yoga. The thumb is folded over to the base of the ring finger, and the other four fingers are closed over it to form a fist. See the second Lungsang for a demonstration of a vajra fist.

wind: In the context of Tibetan medicine, *wind* can either refer to one of the five elements (also called air in this context, along with earth, water, fire, and space) or one of the three energies (in the triad consisting of wind, bile, and phlegm energy). The Tibetan term, *lung,* can also refer more generally to our physical breath and the essence of life itself—our energy, power, life force. See also *elements, five; pranas, five;* and *wind energy.*

wind energy: In Tibetan medicine, one of the three humors or energies that form the basis for the functioning of the human body. Wind energy is first and foremost the life force that is inseparable from the mind of the individual. It is both the air we breathe and our internal energy. Residing in specific areas of the body such as the brain and nerves, heart and chest, digestive tract and anal region, as well as in the bones, wind energy governs many functions of body and mind, in particular those having to do with motility. Memory, awareness, sense perception, speech, physical movements, the generation of effort, the opening and closing of the orifices, the workings of the nervous system, and the circulation of the nutritive essence through blood all depend on wind energy. The Tibetan term for wind energy is *lung*. Ayurveda uses the Sanskrit word *vata*. See also *energies, three* and *pranas, five*.

Yantra: Sanskrit term that literally means "instrument" or "machine" but commonly referring to a geometric figure whose shape is considered a suitable instrument or medium to provoke a meditative experience. In the context of Yantra Yoga, it mainly refers to the movement of the body. The Tibetan term is *trulkhor*.

Yantra Yoga: An ancient tradition of yoga brought to Tibet by the legendary Buddhist master Padmasambhava and preserved in its original and unadulterated form since the eighth century. While some positions look similar to the asanas of Indian traditions such as Hatha Yoga, they are applied in a different way since the main emphasis is on the correct shaping of the breathing rather than on the position itself. Other aspects of the practice, such as the three preliminary groups, are also unique. Yantra Yoga consists of three groups of preliminary exercises, five series of Yantra exercises, and a number of pranayamas. A key focus is the coordination of breathing and movement based on a specific rhythm. Yantra Yoga was originally kept secret and was taught and practiced as a means to deepen and support spiritual realization.

Chögyal Namkhai Norbu, an eminent Tibetan scholar and Dzogchen master, began to teach Yantra Yoga to Western students in the early 1970s, when he was a professor of Tibetan and Mongolian language at the Institute of Oriental Studies at the University of Naples. Over the decades, the number of practitioners has multiplied. Courses are taught all over the world by a growing number of instructors accredited in a rigorous training and examination process.

For more information, visit www.yantrayoga.org.

Further Reading and Resources

Yantra Yoga: The Tibetan Yoga of Movement. By Chögyal Namkhai Norbu, translated by Adriano Clemente. Ithaca, NY: Snow Lion Publications, 2008. Comprehensive manual of the practice of Yantra Yoga, including a translation of Vairochana's eighth-century Union of the Sun and Moon Yantra and the author's extensive commentary.

Rainbow Body: The Life and Realization of Togden Ugyen Tendzin. By Chögyal Namkhai Norbu, translated by Adriano Clemente. Arcidosso, Italy: Shang Shung Publications, 2010. Biography of Tibetan yogin Togden Ugyen Tendzin (1888–1962), who taught Yantra Yoga to Chögyal Namkhai Norbu.

The Crystal and the Way of Light: Sutra, Tantra, and Dzogchen. By Chögyal Namkhai Norbu, edited by John Shane. Ithaca, NY: Snow Lion Publications, 1999. A description of the spiritual path from the viewpoint of Dzogchen against the backdrop of a fascinating autobiographical narrative.

Dzogchen Teachings. By Chögyal Namkhai Norbu. Ithaca, NY: Snow Lion Publications, 2006. Collection of teachings on the basic principles of Dzogchen.

Birth, Life, and Death. By Chögyal Namkhai Norbu, translated by Elio Guarisco. Arcidosso, Italy: Shang Shung Publications, 2008. Basic principles of Tibetan traditional medicine.

Healing with Fire: A Practical Manual of Tibetan Moxibustion. By Chögyal Namkhai Norbu, translated by Elio Guarisco. Arcidosso, Italy: Shang Shung Publications, 2011. Practical guide to the practice of moxibustion from the perspective of Tibetan medicine.

DVDs

Tibetan Yoga of Movement: Level One. Two DVDs with senior instructors Fabio Andrico and Laura Evangelisti together with other Yantra Yoga practitioners. Arcidosso, Italy: Shang Shung Publications, 2011. Movements covered in Level One: Vairochana Posture; Warm-Ups; Nine Purification Breathings; Tsigjong: Loosening the Joints; Lungsang: Purifying the Prana; Tsadul: Controlling the Energy Channels; The Five Yantras of the First Series; Vajra Wave: Overcoming Energy Obstacles.

Tibetan Yoga of Movement: Level Two. Two DVDs with senior instructors Fabio Andrico and Laura Evangelisti together with other Yantra Yoga practitioners. Arcidosso, Italy: Shang Shung Publications, 2011. Movements covered in Level Two: Five Yantras of the Second Series; Five Yantras of the Third Series; Five Yantras of the Fourth Series; Five Yantras of the Fifth Series; Rhythmic Breathing: Pranayama; Vajra Wave: Overcoming Energy Obstacles.

breAthe: The Perfect Harmony of Breathing. DVD with Fabio Andrico and Yamila Diaz. Arcidosso, Italy: Shang Shung Publications, 2011. Simple but effective exercises to deepen and clarify the experience of breathing. Suitable for all levels.

My Reincarnation. DVD. Directed by Jennifer Fox. Coproduction of Zohe Film Productions, Buddhist Broadcasting Foundation, Lichtblick Film, Ventura Film, and Vivo Film, 2010. Feature-length biographical documentary shot over a twenty-year period following Tibetan spiritual master Chögyal Namkhai Norbu and his Italian-born son, Yeshi Silvano Namkhai (Khyentse Yeshe).

Websites

Official Yantra Yoga website
  (including list of authorized instructors):
  www.yantrayoga.org
Dzogchen Community:
  www.tsegyalgar.org (North America)
  www.dzogchen.it (Western Europe)
  www.dzogchen.ro (Eastern Europe)
  www.dzogchen.org.au (Oceania and Australia)
  www.dzogchencommunity.ru (Russia and Ukraine)
  www.tashigarnorte.org (Venezuela)
  www.tashigarsur.com (Argentina)
DzogchenTV YouTube channel:
  www.youtube.com/user/dzogchentv
Shang Shung Institute:
  www.shangshunginstitute.org
Shang Shung Publications:
  www.shangshungpublications.org
  www.shangshungstore.org

Index of Health Benefits

THIS INDEX IDENTIFIES conditions, body parts, pranas, elements, and energies benefited by specific Yantras or preliminary group exercises. Refer to the glossary of terms for attributes related to individual pranas and elements. Certain benefits, such as improved breathing capacity or quality, joint flexibility, and vitality in general, are attributed to specific exercises even though they are also a result of the practice of Yantra Yoga as a whole.

Abdominal bloating: the Dog

Agitation, anxiety (see also *life-sustaining prana*): 6th Lungsang, the Frog, pranayamas in general

Appetite, lack of: the Curved Knife, the Bow

Arms: 2nd Lungsang, 3rd Tsadul, the Dagger, the Eagle

Arthritis: the Conch

Ascending prana (see also *pranas, five*): 5th Lungsang, 6th Lungsang, 3rd Tsadul, 5th Tsadul, the Camel, the Flame, the Vulture, the Dove, the Trident

Asthma (see also *life-sustaining prana*): the Curved Knife

Back: see *spine and spinal cord*

Bile energy: the Jewel, the Sword

Blood energy: the Turtle

Brain: 6th Lungsang, the Sword

Calculi: the Spider

Chest (see also *thoracic region*): 3rd Tsadul, the Turtle, the Frog

Cold-nature disorders: the Conch, the Spider

Depression (see also *life-sustaining prana*): 6th Lungsang, the Half-Moon

Kidneys (see also *organs, solid*): 3rd Tsigjong, 4th Tsigjong, the Camel, the Conch, the Curved Knife, the Dog, the Spider, the Bow, the Eagle

Large intestine (see also *organs, hollow*): the Dog, the Locust, the Tiger

Legs: 4th Tsigjong, 2nd Tsadul, the Dagger, the Eagle

Life-sustaining prana (see also *pranas, five*): 6th Lungsang, the Frog, all pranayamas, all five series of Yantras in general

Ligaments: 2nd Tsigjong, 3rd Tsigjong, 4th Lungsang, 3rd Tsadul (of the arms and shoulders), 4th Tsadul (of the shoulders), the Conch (of the lumbar region), the Plow (of the head and limbs), the Snake (of the head and limbs), the Dagger (of the head and limbs), the Dog, the Bow, the Triangle (of the head and limbs), the Tiger (of the head and limbs)

Limbs (see also *pervasive prana*): 5th Tsigjong (sensory-motor dysfunctions of), 2nd Lungsang, the Plow (ligaments of), the Snake (ligaments of), the Bow (ligaments and tendons of), the Triangle (muscles, ligaments, and tendons of), the Locust (lower, loss of sensation in), the Tiger (nerves and ligaments of), the Wheel (muscles and tendons of), the Frog (joints, tendons, and muscles of)

Liver (see also *organs, solid*): the Conch, the Turtle, the Half-Moon, the Frog

Lower body, functions of: 3rd Tsigjong

Lucidity: 1st Lungsang, the Lion, the Sword

Lumbar region: 3rd Tsigjong, 4th Tsigjong, 3rd Lungsang, the Camel, the Conch, the Flame, the Curved Knife, the Spider, the Bow, the Half-Moon, the Locust, the Wheel, the Eagle

Lungs (see also *organs, solid*): 5th Lungsang, 4th Tsadul

Lymph (see also *elements, five*): 1st Tsadul

Memory (see also *ascending prana*): 6th Lungsang

Stomach mucus, accumulation of: the Curved Knife

Nerves (see also *pervasive prana*): 6th Lungsang (of the sense organs), 4th Tsadul (of the shoulders), the Turtle (of the solid and hollow organs), the Vulture (of the solid and sense organs), the Tiger (of the head and limbs), the Sword (of the sense organs and brain), the Peacock (of the solid and hollow organs)

Neurological disorders: 2nd Lungsang

Neuromuscular functions: the Lion

Numbness: the Flame

Organs, hollow (stomach, small intestine, large intestine, gallbladder, urinary bladder, and seminal vesicles or ovaries): 3rd Lungsang, 4th

Lungsang, 7th Lungsang, 8th Lungsang, 5th Tsadul, the Camel, the Conch, the Turtle, the Plow, the Snake, the Bow, the Half-Moon, the Lion, the Triangle, the Peacock

Organs, solid (heart, lungs, liver, spleen, and kidneys): 1st Lungsang, 3rd Lungsang, 4th Lungsang, 8th Lungsang, the Camel, the Turtle, the Plow, the Snake, the Spider, the Bow, the Half-Moon, the Lion, the Vulture, the Triangle, the Peacock

Ovaries: see *organs, hollow*

Pain in the joints and muscles, diffuse: the Lion

Pelvis: the Camel

Pervasive prana (see also *pranas, five*): 1st Tsigjong, 5th Tsigjong, 4th Lungsang, 5th Lungsang, 1st Tsadul, the Dog, the Locust, the Dove, the Wheel

Phlegm energy: the Conch, the Turtle, the Curved Knife, the Dove, the Jewel, the Sword

Physical condition and vitality in general: 1st Tsigjong, 1st Lungsang

Prana and breathing in general: the Nine Purification Breathings, all pranayamas, Lungsangs in general

Pranas, five (see also under the individual pranas): the Plow, the Snake, the Spider, the Bow, the Half-Moon, the Lion, the Vulture, the Triangle, the Trident, the Jewel, the Eagle, the Sword, the Peacock, all five series of Yantras in general, in particular for life-sustaining prana

Reproductive functions (see also *downward-clearing prana*): 3rd Tsigjong

Respiratory problems: the Curved Knife

Rib cage: 3rd Lungsang, 4th Tsadul, the Half-Moon

Sciatica: the Flame, the Locust, the Tiger, the Wheel

Seminal vesicles: see *organs, hollow*

Senses, five: 1st Tsigjong, 6th Lungsang, the Vulture, the Eagle, the Sword, all five series of Yantras in general

Sensory-motor coordination: 5th Tsigjong

Shoulders: 2nd Lungsang, 3rd Tsadul, 4th Tsadul, the Dove

Skin: 1st Tsadul

Small intestine (see also *organs, hollow*): the Dog, the Locust, the Tiger

Spine and spinal cord: 4th Tsigjong, 3rd Lungsang, 5th Lungsang, 7th Lungsang, 5th Tsadul, the Camel, the Flame, the Plow, the Snake, the Dog, the Bow, the Triangle, the Tiger, the Wheel, the Eagle, the Frog

Spleen: see *organs, solid*

Stiffness: 5th Tsigjong, the Tiger, the Wheel

Stomach (see also *organs, hollow*): the Tiger

Strength, physical: the Dagger, the Jewel, the Eagle, all five series of Yantras in general

Tendons: 4th Tsigjong (of the legs), 4th Lungsang, 2nd Tsadul (of the feet and legs), the Dagger (of the head and limbs), the Dog, the Bow, the Triangle (of the head and limbs), the Wheel (of the head and limbs), the Frog (of the head and limbs)

Thoracic region (see also *life-sustaining prana*): 4th Tsigjong, 2nd Lungsang

Tingling: the Flame

Torso: the Dagger, the Bow, the Dove

Ulcers: the Turtle

Urinary bladder: see *organs, hollow*

Waist area (see also *Lumbar region*): 3rd Lungsang

Wind energy: 4th Lungsang, 1st Tsadul, the Flame, the Jewel, the Wheel, the Sword

About the Authors

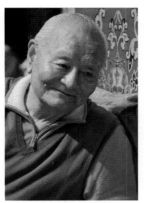

BORN IN EASTERN Tibet in 1938, **Chögyal Namkhai Norbu** is an internationally known Dzogchen Buddhist teacher and author as well as an eminent scholar of the culture of Tibet. During his childhood and youth, he received many teachings from renowned masters of various Tibetan Buddhist traditions. In the 1960s, he was invited to collaborate with leading Tibetologist Giuseppe Tucci in Italy and about a decade later began to give instructions to Western students on the practice of Yantra Yoga and Dzogchen Buddhism. He is the author of *Yantra Yoga: The Tibetan Yoga of Movement* and many other books on Tibetan culture and Dzogchen as well as the founder of ASIA and the Shang Shung Institute, two nonprofit organizations dedicated to supporting the Tibetan people and preserving Tibetan culture.

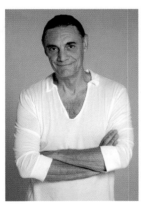

Born and raised in Italy, **Fabio Andrico** is an internationally recognized expert on Yantra Yoga. He is one of the closest students of the great Dzogchen master Chögyal Namkhai Norbu, who introduced Yantra Yoga to the West in the early 1970s. Andrico, who initially studied Hatha Yoga in India, has been learning, practicing, teaching, and writing about Yantra Yoga since the late 1970s. He regularly conducts courses, workswhops, and teacher trainings around the world, including Kripalu, Esalen, and Yoga Tree in the USA and Yoga Federation in Russia, and has appeared in yoga DVDs such as *The Eight Movements of Yantra Yoga*, *BreAthe*, and *Tibetan Yoga of Movement, Levels 1 and 2*. He also collaborated on the book *Yantra Yoga: The Tibetan Yoga of Movement*.